Manual on

Postpartum Hemorrhage

68th All India Congress of Obstetrics & Gynaecology

aicog Delhi 2026

Advocate Innovate Challenge Optimise Globalise

Manual on
Postpartum Hemorrhage

Series Editors

Ashok Kumar
MD PhD
Director–Professor
Department of Obstetrics and Gynecology
Atal Bihari Vajpayee Institute of Medical Sciences
and Dr Ram Manohar Lohia Hospital
New Delhi, India

Madhavi M Gupta
MS
Director–Professor
Department of Obstetrics and Gynecology
Maulana Azad Medical College and Lok Nayak Hospital
New Delhi, India

K Aparna Sharma
MBBS MD
Professor
Department of Obstetrics and Gynecology
All India Institute of Medical Sciences
New Delhi, India

Editors

Manju Puri
Rashmi Kahar
Charmila Ayyavoo
Reena Rani Punia

Co-Editors

Deepti Gupta
Padma Shukla
Mahesh Gupta
Ruby Bhatia

JAYPEE

JAYPEE BROTHERS MEDICAL PUBLISHERS
The Health Sciences Publisher
New Delhi | London

Message from Series Editors

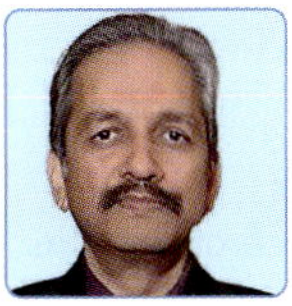

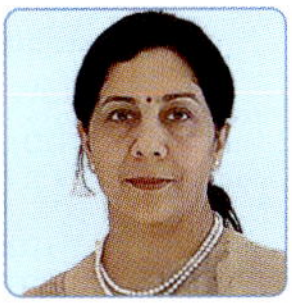

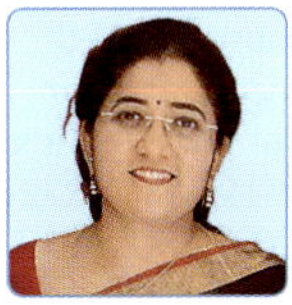

Ashok Kumar
Organizing Chairperson
AICOG-2026
New Delhi

Madhavi M Gupta
Organizing Secretary
AICOG-2026
New Delhi

K Aparna Sharma
Organizing Secretary
AICOG-2026
New Delhi

It is after 18 long years that the 68th AICOG is being held in New Delhi. It is a pleasure to welcome you all.

The Organizing Team have poured their heart and soul into curating an academic program which one will feel a loss if missed. The scientific sessions include both national and international faculty who are stalwarts in their fields. There are 18 workshops with 8 full-day and 5 each in the pre-lunch and post-lunch time.

On this occasion, the workshop faculty, have gone that extra mile to publish the workshop manual for eight workshops. This includes all recent scientific evidence and clinical management guidelines. These manuals will serve as a go-to evidence-based resource in your day-to-day clinical practice. We look forward to receiving your valuable feedback.

We acknowledge the hard work put in by all the editors, co-editors, and the authors, who, in spite of busy schedules and time constraints, have contributed immensely.

We would also like to thank M/s Jaypee Brothers Medical Publishers (P) Ltd, New Delhi, India, for partnering with us.

We sincerely hope that you will enjoy reading these manuals, find this manual useful, and treasure it for future use in your practical work.

We take this opportunity to wish you a memorable time during your stay in New Delhi.

Warm Regards

JAYPEE **Jaypee Brothers Medical Publishers (P) Ltd**

Headquarters
EMCA House, 23/23-B
Ansari Road, Daryaganj
New Delhi 110 002, India
Landline: +91-11-23272143, +91-11-23272703
+91-11-23282021, +91-11-23245672
e-mail: jaypee@jaypeebrothers.com

Corporate Office
4838/24, Ansari Road, Daryaganj
New Delhi 110 002, India
Phone: +91-11-43574357
Fax: +91-11-43574314
e-mail: jaypee@jaypeebrothers.com

Overseas Office
JP Medical Ltd.
83, Victoria Street, London
SW1H 0HW (UK)
Phone: +44-20 3170 8910
e-mail: info@jpmedpub.com

EU GPSR Authorised Representative
Logos Europe, 9 rue Nicolas Poussin
17000, La Rochelle, France
Phone: +33 (0) 6 67 93 73 78
e-mail: contact@logoseurope.eu

Website: www.jaypeebrothers.com
Website: www.jaypeedigital.com

Inquiries for bulk sales may be solicited at: jaypee@jaypeebrothers.com

Manual on Postpartum Hemorrhage

First Edition: **2026**

ISBN: 978-93-7545-055-9

Printed at: Samrat Offset Pvt. Ltd.

Contributors

Aditi Rathore MS FICOG
Consultant
Rathore Nursing Home
Ratlam, Madhya Pradesh, India

Ami Surti MBBS DGO DNB
Consultant
Department of Obstetrics
and Gynecology
Surya Group of Hospitals
Mumbai, Maharashtra, India

Ashish Narendra Zarariya MBBS MD
Associate Professor
Department of Obstetrics
and Gynecology
Government Medical College
and Hospital
Nagpur, Maharashtra, India

Ashwin Rao
MBBS MS FRM FMAS FARIS PGDMLS
Consultant Reproductive Medicine,
Endogynecology and Robotics
Salem Polyclinic
Salem, Tamil Nadu, India

Chandrakala Maran
DNB (Obs & Gyne)
Head
Department of Obstetrics
and Gynecology
KG Hospital and Postgraduate Institute
Coimbatore, Tamil Nadu, India

Charmila Ayyavoo
MD DGO DFP FICOG PGDCR
Assistant Professor
Dhanalakshmi Srinivasan
Medical College
Perambalur, Tamil Nadu, India
Aditi Hospital, Aditi Pluro-Fertility Center
Tiruchirappalli, Tamil Nadu

Deepti Gupta
MBBS MS DNB FICOG FMAS
Associate Professor
Department of Obstetrics
and Gynecology
Netaji Subhash Chandra Bose
Medical College, Jabalpur
Consultant and Unit Head
Ankur Fertility Clinic and IVF Center
Jabalpur, Madhya Pradesh, India

Ishika Nain MS
Consultant and Laparoscopic Surgeon
Sapra Multispeciality Hospital
Hisar, Haryana, India
Secretary HOGS 2020

Jaya Tulaskar MS DRM MCOG
Consultant (Obstetrics
and Gynecology)
Tulaskar Hospital
Wardha, Maharashtra, India

Kena Gandhi MBBS MD
Junior Resident
Department of Obstetrics
and Gynecology
SGT Medical College
Gurugram, Haryana, India

Kiran Chandna
MBBS DGO FICOG PGDUSG
Senior Consultant and Director
Chandna Medical Centre
Faridabad, Haryana, India

Kirtan M Vyas MBBS MS FICOG
Consultant and Director
Department of Obstetrics and
Gynecology
Sevak Maternity and Surgical Hospital
Ahmedabad, Gujarat, India

Komal Bansal MBBS
Senior Resident
Department of Obstetrics
and Gynecology
Maharishi Markandeshwar Institute
of Medical Sciences and Research
Mullana, Ambala, Haryana, India

Komal Yadav MBBS
Postgraduate Student
Department of Obstetrics
and Gynecology
Maulana Azad Medical College
New Delhi, India

Mahak Singaal
Assistant Professor
Department of Obstetrics
and Gynecology
Maharishi Markandeshwar Institute
of Medical Sciences and
Research Mullana
Ambala, Haryana, India

Mahesh Gupta MD
Department of Obstetrics
and Gynecology
Pushpam Hospital
Ahmedabad, Gujarat, India

Manju Puri MBBS MD
Professor
Department of Obstetrics
and Gynecology
SGT Medical College
Gurugram, Haryana, India

Megha Karnik
MS DNB FMAS
Assistant Professor
Department of Obstetrics
and Gynecology
Jawaharlal Nehru Medical College
Wardha, Maharashtra, India

Munjal J Pandya MS (Obs & Gyne)
Associate Professor
Narendra Modi Medical College
Ahmedabad, Gujarat, India

Nitu Mishra MS DNB MNAMS
Associate Professor
Department of Obstetrics
and Gynecology
All India Institute of Medical Sciences
Bhopal, Madhya Pradesh, India

Padma Shukla MS FICOG FICMCH
Associate Professor
Department of Obstetrics
and Gynecology
Shyam Shah Medical College (SSMC)
Rewa, Madhya Pradesh, India

Poorva Badkur MS
Assistant Professor
Department of Obstetrics
and Gynecology
Gandhi Medical College
Bhopal, Madhya Pradesh, India

Priyanshi Nigam MBBS
Senior Resident
Shyam Shah Medical College (SSMC)
Rewa, Madhya Pradesh, India

Rajasi Kane Sengupta
MBBS MD DNB FICOG
Professor and Head
Department of Obstetrics
and Gynecology
Datta Meghe Medical College
Nagpur, Maharashtra, India

Rashmi Kahar
MBBS DGO FICOG FICMCH MCOG
Senior Consultant (Obstetrics
and Gynecology)
Dr Rajendra Gode Medical College
Amravati, Maharashtra, India
Director, Kharodkar Hospital
Amravati, Maharashtra, India
Chairperson, FOGSI Practical Obstetrics
Committee 2025–2027

Reena Rani Punia MS MRCOG DNB FCLS
Assistant Professor
Department of Obstetrics
and Gynecology
Maulana Azad Medical College
New Delhi, India

Ruby Bhatia MD MS
Professor and Head
Department of Obstetrics
and Gynecology
Maharishi Markandeshwar Institute
of Medical Sciences and Research
Mullana, Ambala, Haryana, India

Samartha Ram H MBBS DGO
Head
Sandhya Ram Maternity Hospital
Palakkad, Kerala, India

Shalini V Singh MBBS MD DNB FMAS
Assistant Professor
Department of Obstetrics
and Gynecology
Dr Ram Manohar Lohia Institute
of Medical Sciences
Lucknow, Uttar Pradesh, India

Shashi L Kabra Maheshwari
MD FICOG FMAS
Consultant (SAG)
Department of Obstetrics
and Gynecology
DDU Hospital, Govt of NCT
New Delhi, India

Shuchi Sehgal MBBS MD
Senior Resident
Department of Obstetrics
and Gynecology
Netaji Subhash Chandra Bose
Medical College
Jabalpur, Madhya Pradesh, India

Sruthi AV MBBS DNB FMAS DMAS
Consultant
Department of Obstetrics
and Gynecology
Sandhya Ram Maternity Hospital
Palakkad, Kerala, India

Suchitra N Pandit
MBBS MD DNB FRCOG (UK) FICOG DFP
BPharm
Senior Consultant
Department of Obstetrics
and Gynecology
Surya Group of Hospitals
Mumbai, Maharashtra, India
FOGSI Representative to
FIGO (2026-28)
FOGSI Representative to
SAFOG (2023–2025)
Member FIGO Ethics
Committee (2025–2027)
Chair AICC RCOG (2018–2020)
President FOGSI & ICOG (2014–2015)

VP Paily MD FRGOG
Senior Consultant
Department of Obstetrics
and Gynecology
Rajagiri Hospital
Aluva, Kerala, India

Preface

Postpartum Hemorrhage remains a leading cause of maternal mortality and morbidity worldwide. It continues to present us a significant challenge. There are disparities in the care provided, its implementation and quality. The Sustainable Development Goal for maternal mortality ratio set by the United Nations for 2030 seems tangible and attainable. It has been a remarkable trend of decline in maternal mortality ratio. However, there is a huge discrepancy in performance of various states with the 9 Empowered Action Group States and Assam still having a maternal mortality ratio of 137 per 100000 live births. Improving awareness and hence interventions in control and management of postpartum hemorrhage can go a long way in saving maternal lives.

This manual is intended to provide basic and advanced updates on the subject. It conglomerates evidences on pathophysiology, prevention and management of postpartum hemorrhage. Particular attention has been given to interactions between system-level determinants, like skills and drills, referral services, and point-of-care services.

It also examines the effectiveness, feasibility of interventions like active management of third stage of labor, uterotonics, non-pneumatic antishock garment, and surgical-nonsurgical procedures in diverse settings (WHO, FIGO)

This book highlights the medical and surgical management of postpartum hemorrhage. Many untouched areas like retained placenta, lacunae in estimation of blood loss have been clarified and role of newer modern inventions, newer modalities and newer guidelines on *Postpartum hemorrhage* have been elucidated. This manual covers analysis of why mothers die of hemorrhage and proposed preventive strategies. It is truly a manual for every practicing obstetrician to help maximize the golden hour.

Editors: **Manju Puri, Rashmi Kahar, Charmila Ayyavoo, Reena Rani Punia**

Co-Editors: **Deepti Gupta, Padma Shukla, Mahesh Gupta, Ruby Bhatia**

Contents

1 CHAPTER

Overview of Postpartum Hemorrhage

Megha Karnik, Rashmi Kahar

INTRODUCTION

Maternal mortality is defined as the death of any woman from complications arising during or aggravated due to pregnancy, irrespective of the duration and site of pregnancy, childbirth, or within 42 days of termination of pregnancy, excluding incidental or accidental causes. Maternal mortality is measured through maternal mortality ratio (MMR), which is defined as the number of maternal deaths per 100,000 live births. The **Figure 1** shows the global MMR for the year 2020.

At a MMR of 97 per 100,000 live births in 2020, India still contributed to 8.3% (24,000) of maternal deaths. Within the country the MMR varies between the various states, with Kerla having the lowest MMR of 19 and Assam having the highest MMR of 195 **(Fig. 2)**.

The leading causes of maternal mortality in India are Postpartum hemorrhage (47%), Sepsis and infections (12%) and hypertensive disorders of pregnancy (7%) as depicted in **Figure 3**.

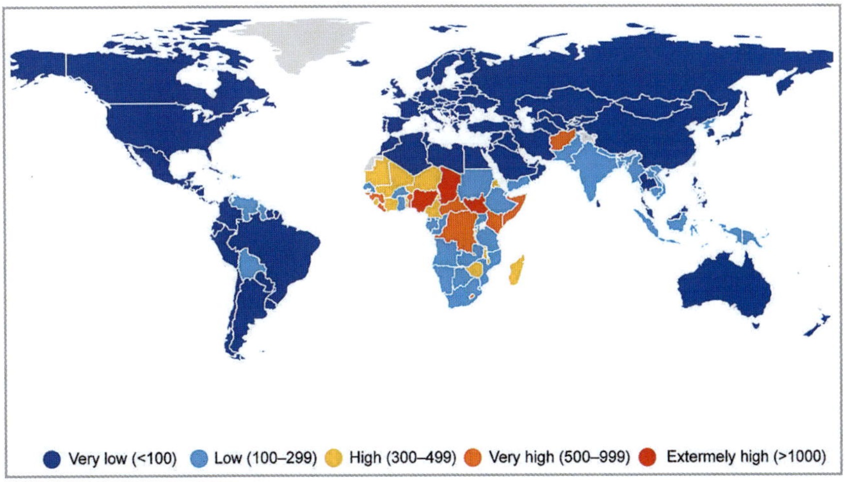

Fig. 1: Global MMR 2020.
Source: World Health Organization, UNICEF, United Nations Population Fund and The World Bank. Trends in Maternal Mortality: 2000 to 2020 WHO: Geneva, 2023.

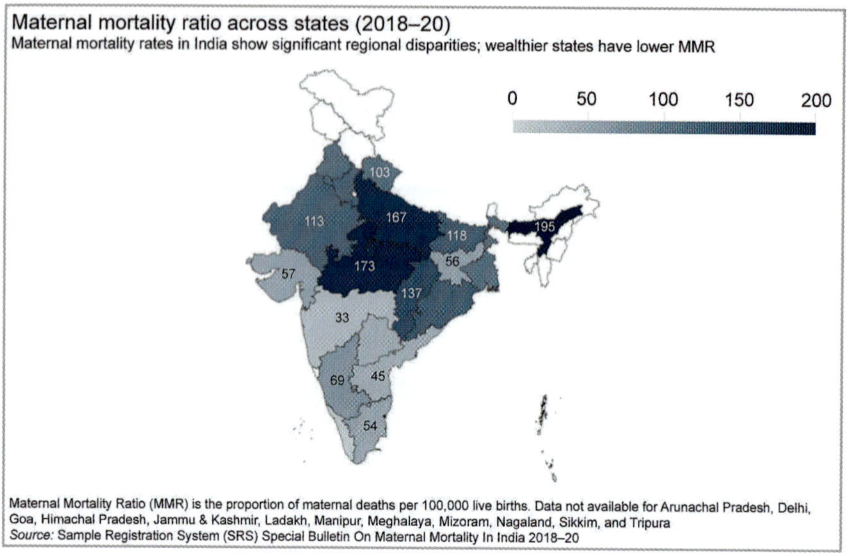

Fig. 2: Maternal mortality ratio across states in India 2020.

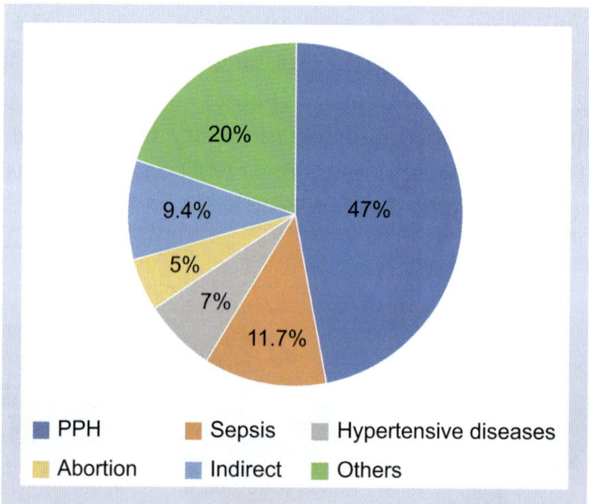

Fig. 3: Causes of maternal deaths in India 2020.
Source: Meh C, Sharma A, Ram U, Fadel S, Correa N, Snelgrove JW, et al. Trends in maternal mortality in India over two decades in nationally representative surveys. BJOG. 2022;129(4):550-61.

POSTPARTUM HEMORRHAGE: DEFINITION

As per the latest definition for PPH by WHO (2012), PPH is defined as a blood loss of 500 mL or more within 24 hours after a vaginal birth and 1,000 mL after a cesarean section, while severe PPH is defined as a blood loss of 1,000 mL or more within the same timeframe. National Health Mission, India defines

Postpartum Hemorrhage (PPH) is commonly defined as a blood loss of 500 mL or more within 24 hours after birth, or a small blood loss that makes the woman hemodynamically unstable is also termed as PPH. Massive/severe PPH is defined as a blood loss of 1,000 mL or more within the same timeframe. Hemorrhage between 24 hours and 6 weeks postpartum is termed "delayed PPH."

However, the above definitions do not take into account the hemodynamic status and reserve of the woman. The modified shock index can be a clinical marker of PPH and clinical outcomes. The MSI is defined as heart rate (HR) to mean arterial pressure (MAP). MAP is measured by the formula: $MAP = DP + 1/3(SP - DP)$ or $MAP = DP + 1/3(PP)$. The normal range varies between 0.5–0.7 in healthy adults. The MSI may have prognostic importance and also serves as a guide for the type of interventions required in the management of PPH **(Table 1)**.

Risk Factors for PPH

Every pregnancy has an inherent risk of PPH and identification of risk factors in the antenatal period is one of the effective means of preparedness during and after delivery. These risk factors take into account both early and late PPH **(Table 2)**.

Causes of Postpartum Hemorrhage: The 4Ts

The causes of postpartum hemorrhage can be summarized in the 4Ts i.e., Tone, Tissue, Trauma, and Thrombin as summarized in **Figure 4**.

A review of history and physical examination along with per speculum vaginal examination would help in identification of the cause of PPH. examination of the patient at the time of ongoing hemorrhage can help in the identification of the likely cause of bleeding. A boggy, soft uterus is suggestive of atonic uterus. Indentation at the uterine fundus or inability to palpate the uterus may point toward uterine inversion. Similarly, vaginal bleeding with a well retracted uterus prompts vaginal

TABLE 1: Correlation of shock index and interventions.

Status of shock	*Shock index*	*Intervention*
No shock	<0.6	Nil
Mild shock	≥0.6 to <1.0	Iv fluids, medical management
Moderate shock	≥1.0 to <1.4	• ≥1.0 to <1.3: Operative interventions • ≥1.3: ICU admission, massive blood transfusion, and increased morbidity
Severe shock	≥1.4	• Massive blood transfusion protocols • >1.6: associated with mortality

TABLE 2: Risk factors for PPH.

Maternal factors	
• Teenage/Elderly primigravida • Multiparity and Grand multiparity (>4) • Poor antenatal care • Low socioeconomic status • Previous postpartum hemorrhage • Previous uterine surgeries, rupture • Uterine malformations • Fibroid uterus • Previous cesarean section • Anemia • Thrombocytopenia • Diabetes • Cardiac dysfunction	• Hypertensive disorders • Thyroid dysfunction • IVF • Renal and liver disorders • Anticoagulant therapy • Viral infections, dengue • Inherited and acquired coagulopathies • Hemoglobinopathies • Metabolic syndrome • Post-bariatric surgery • Pregnancy after renal transplant • Multifetal gestation
Fetal factors	
• Large-for-gestational-age fetus • Fetal macrosomia (birth weight greater than 4,000 g) • Polyhydramnios	
Placental factors	
• Placenta previa • Placenta abruption • Placenta accreta • AV malformations • Chorioangioma • Placental abnormalities (battle door placenta, vasa previa	
Intrapartum	
• Induction and augmentation of labor • Precipitate labor and prolonged labor • Obstructed labor • The arrest of labor in the second stage • Trial of labor after cesarean (TOLAC)/ vaginal birth after cesarean (VBAC)	• Instrumental deliveries, cesarean section • In-coordinate uterine action (hypotonic and hypertonic) • Prolonged rupture of the membrane (PROM/PPORM) • Chorioamnionitis • Placenta abruption
Postpartum	
• Genital tract trauma • Retained placenta or placental tissues • Uterine inversion, uterine rupture • Subinvolution • Puerperal sepsis	

exploration to rule out traumatic PPH. A slow trickle, or oozing of blood from venepuncture site is likely suggestive of coagulation defect in the absence of uterine atomy and trauma.

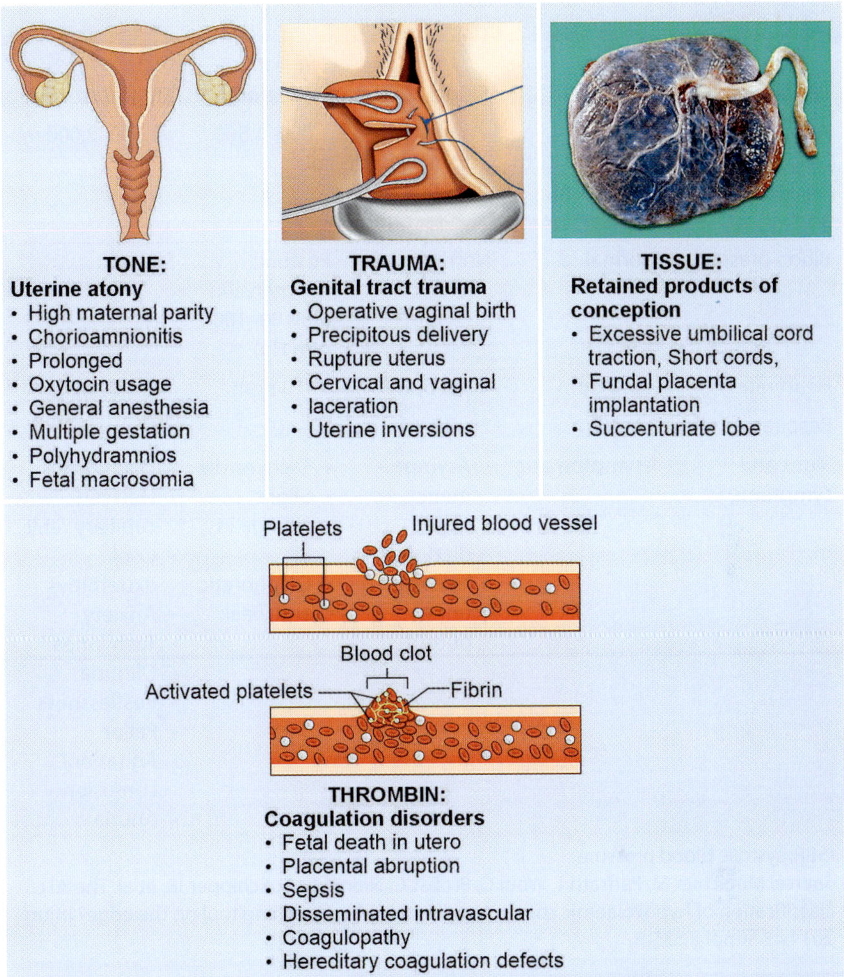

Fig. 4: Causes of postpartum hemorrhage—the 4Ts.

Assessment of Blood Loss

Clinical signs or symptoms of shock, such as tachycardia and hypotension, may be masked in some cases due to physiological changes in pregnancy. While these signs become evident, considerable blood loss of more than 25% may have occurred. It is important that for the safety of the patient, a continuous assessment of the vital signs and an estimation of the ongoing blood loss should be done. The signs of shock can help in the estimation of blood loss **(Table 3)**.

Rapid assessment of blood loss is crucial in the management of PPH. However, accurate assessment of actual blood loss may prove challenging during an emergency as clinicians may over or underestimate the blood loss amount.

TABLE 3: Estimation of blood loss and clinical signs and symptoms.

Parameter	*Stage 0*	*Stage 1 (mild)*	*Stage 2 (moderate)*	*Stage 3 (severe)*
Approximate blood loss	• 500 mL-vaginal birth • 1,000 mL -c-section	• >500 mL-vaginal birth • >1,000 mL -c-section	1,000–1,500 mL	>1,500–2,000 mL
Blood pressure	Normal	Normal	Postural hypotension (SBP 80–100 mm Hg)	SBP <80
Heart rate	<100 bpm	<100 bpm	>110 bpm	>120 bpm
Respiratory rate	14–20	20–30	30–40	>40
Signs and symptoms	Asymptomatic	• Asymptomatic • Slight dizziness • Normal urine output	• Tachycardia • Slight change in BP • Diaphoretic and weak	• Diaphoresis • Delayed capillary refill • Cool extremities • Anxiety • Tachypnea • Oliguria • Restlessness • Pallor • Agitation/ confusion • Anuria

(SBP: systolic blood pressure)
Source: Mutschler M, Paffrath T, Wölfl C, Probst C, Nienaber U, Schipper IB, et al. The ATLS® classification of hypovolaemic shock: A well established teaching tool on the edge? Injury. 2014;45 Suppl 3:S35-8.

Visual estimation of blood loss can be done by measuring the soaked perineal pads, blood collected in drapes and bucket, spillage of blood on the bed or floor, and suction machine (in case of cesarean section) **(Table 4)**. However, these methods can underestimate the extent of blood loss due to its subjective nature. Brass-V Drapes as another rapid too to estimate blood loss.

Investigations in the Management of PPH

A battery of investigations is needed for the management and diagnosis of postpartum hemorrhage. These include:

- Complete blood count and hemoglobin, hematocrit
- *Bed side tests:* Bleeding time, clotting time, clot observation test (in low resource setting)

TABLE 4: Visual estimation of blood loss.

One fully soaked perineal pad	100 mL
Half-soaked perineal pad	60 mL
Less than half soaked pad	30 mL
Fully soaked abdominal mop (45 cm × 45 cm)	150 mL
20 × 20 cm incontinence gauze piece	100 mL
Kelly's pad half soaked	300 mL
Kelly's pad full soaked	500 mL
Full kidney tray	500 mL
Half kidney tray	250 mL
PPH with Blood on bed	1,000 mL
PPH with Floor spill	2,000 mL

Source: Khadilkar SS, Sood A, Ahire P. Quantification of Peri-partum Blood Loss: Training Module and Clot Conversion Factor. J Obstetr Gynecol India. 2016;66(1):307-14.

- Coagulation profile may be deranged in hemorrhagc
  - Bleeding time (BT) increased
  - Clotting time (CT) increased
  - Platelet count (PC) decreased
  - Prothrombin time (PT) increased
  - International normalized ratio (INR) increased in coagulopathy
  - Serum fibrinogen decreased or normal
  - D-Dimers increased
- Serum electrolytes, blood urea, serum creatinine elevated in renal failure, and hemolysis
- *Serum lactate:* Elevated in sepsis
- Serum calcium, magnesium and potassium: Can be low in hemorrhage
- *Ultrasound:* Retained placenta, adherent placenta, inversion, rupture
- *Thromboelastogram (TEG):* Wherever available and feasible
- Arterial blood gas analysis and its interpretation

CURRENT MODALITIES FOR MANAGEMENT OF PPH

PPH is managed at four levels: Zero-hour, medical management, Mechanical management, and surgical management.

a. *Zero hour:* The aim is to secure CABDE response (circulation, airway, breathing, disability, exposure), collection of blood samples, catheterization of bladder, recording of vitals, and shock index.
b. *Medical management:* Palpation of the uterus to rule out atony, vaginal examination for any trauma, manual examination, and bedside ultrasound for retained placental tissue, assessment of blood coagulation disorders,

pharmacological agents (uterotonics, anti-fibrinolytic agents), blood transfusion.

c. *Mechanical management:* Bimanual compression, balloon tamponade, non-pneumatic antishock garment, aortic compression

d. *Surgical management:* Uterine compression sutures, stepwise devascularization, uterine artery embolization, hysterectomy.

Newer approaches to management include the PPH bundle approach, Panikkar's suction cannula and the EMOTIVE bundle.

KEY TAKE-HOME MESSAGES

- PPH is the leading cause of maternal mortality in India despite improvements in MMR; each pregnancy has the potential towards PPH; hence preparedness is the key to management.
- Irrespective of the traditional definition of PPH, it is important to keep in mind the woman's hemodynamic status and Modified Shock index (MSI) over the volume loss alone.
- Continuous monitoring of vitals, estimation of blood loss by various techniques, and rapidly identifying the cause of PPH is imperative to prevent morbidity and mortality.
- Risk assessment should be done in the ante-natal period for birth preparedness and timely referral to higher centers.
- Objective tools such as visual estimation aids, calibrated drapes, vitals, MSI should be used at all times.
- Multidisciplinary teamwork, PPH bundles and standardized protocols (e.g., EMOTIVE bundle) improve response time, reduce morbidity, and mortality.

SUGGESTED READING

1. Abecassis A, Wainstock T, Sheiner E, Miodownik S, Pariente G. Risk factors for early postpartum hemorrhage: A retrospective, population-based, cohort analysis. Int J Gynecol Obstet. 2024;166:812-8.
2. Agarwal V, Suri J, Agarwal P, Gupta S, Mishra PK. Shock Index as a predictor of maternal outcome in postpartum hemorrhage. J South Asian Feder Obs Gynae. 2021;13(3):131-6.
3. Bohren MA, Lorencatto F, Coomarasamy A, Althabe F, Devall AJ, Evans C, et al. Formative research to design an implementation strategy for a postpartum hemorrhage initial response treatment bundle (E-MOTIVE): study protocol. Reprod Health. 2021;18(1):149.
4. Chandraharan E, Krishna A. Diagnosis and management of postpartum haemorrhage. BMJ. 2017;358:j3875.
5. Elbohoty AE, Mohammed WE, Sweed M, Bahaa Eldin AM, Nabhan A, Abd-El-Maeboud KH. Randomized controlled trial comparing carbetocin, misoprostol, and oxytocin for the prevention of postpartum haemorrhage following an elective cesarean delivery. Int J Gynaecol Obstet. 2016;134(3):324-8.
6. Esau J, Morris T, Muller C, Els C, de Waard L. Two Postpartum Blood Collection Devices: The Brass-V Drape and MaternaWell Tray-As Experienced by Birth Attendants and Birthing Women-A Questionnaire-Based Randomised Study. Obstet Gynecol Int. 2024;2024:6605833.

7. Evensen A, Anderson JM, Fontaine P. Postpartum hemorrhage: prevention and treatment. Am Fam Physician. 2017;95(7):442-9.
8. Federation of Obstetrics and Gynecological Society of India. (2022). PPH Prevention and Management: Updated PPH Guidelines 2022. [online] Available from https://www.fogsi.org/wp-content/uploads/tog/pph prevention-and-management-updated-sept-2022.pdf [Last accessed December, 2025].
9. Goli S, Puri P, Salve PS, Pallikadavath S, James KS. Estimates and correlates of district-level maternal mortality ratio in India. PLOS Glob Public Health. 2022;2(7):e0000441.
10. Hoveyda F, MacKenzie IZ. Secondary postpartum haemorrhage: Incidence, morbidity management. BJOG. 2001;108(9): 927-30.
11. Khadilkar SS, Sood A, Ahire P. Quantification of Peri-partum Blood Loss: Training Module and Clot Conversion Factor. J Obstetr Gynecol India. 2016; 66(1):307-14.
12. Maternal Health Division Ministry of Health and Family Welfare Government of India. (2015). Guidance Note on Prevention and Management of Postpartum Haemorrhage. [online] Available from https://nhm.gov.in/images/pdf/programmes/maternal-health/guidelines/Guidance_Note_on_Prevention_&_Management_of_Postpartum_Haemorrhage.pdf [Last accessed December,, 2025].
13. Mavrides E, Allard S, Chandraharan E, Collins P, Green L, Hunt BJ, et al ; Royal College of Obstetricians and Gynaecologists. Prevention and management of postpartum haemorrhage. BJOG. 2016;124:e106-49.
14. Meh C, Sharma A, Ram U, Fadel S, Correa N, Snelgrove JW, et al. Trends in maternal mortality in India over two decades in nationally representative surveys. BJOG. 2022;129(4):550-61.
15. Mutschler M, Paffrath T, Wölfl C, Probst C, Nienaber U, Schipper IB, et al. The ATLS® classification of hypovolaemic shock: A well established teaching tool on the edge? et al. Injury. 2014;45 Suppl 3:S35-8.
16. Office of the Registrar General and Census Commissioner, India (ORGI). (2022). Sample Registration System (SRS)-Special Bulletin on Maternal Mortality in India 2018-20. [online] Available from https://censusindia.gov.in/nada/index.php/catalog/44379 [Last accessed December, 2025].
17. WHO, UNICEF, UNFPA, World Bank Group and UNDESA/Population Division. Trends in maternal mortality 2000 to 2020. Geneva: World Health Organization; 2023.
18. World Health Organization, UNICEF, United Nations Population Fund and The World Bank. Trends in Maternal Mortality: 2000 to 2020. Geneva: WHO; 2023.
19. World Health Organization recommendations for the prevention and treatment of postpartum haemorrhage. Geneva: WHO; 2012.

2 CHAPTER

Different Approaches to Blood Loss Estimation in Postpartum Hemorrhage: A Review

Reena Rani Punia, Komal Yadav

INTRODUCTION

Postpartum hemorrhage (PPH) is a leading cause of maternal mortality in developing developed countries. It not only contributes substantially to social and economic burden but also define the health infrastructure of a country. Imperatively, 54–90% of the mortality due to PPH is preventable. Lack of recognition of PPH and delayed activation of PPH treatment bundle can lead to worsening of maternal shock. Blood loss during childbirth is often underestimated especially when blood loss is more than 500 mL. Underestimation leads to delays in diagnosing PPH and suboptimal initiation of life saving interventions resulting in increased risks of morbidity and mortality. Accurate and timely estimation of blood loss is therefore an unmet clinical need and remains central to preventing adverse outcomes associated with PPH. Although overestimation of blood loss is uncommon, when it does occur, it may lead to unnecessary interventions and wastage of limited resources.

FIGO recommend strategies like—Readiness, Recognition, Response, Reporting and Respectful, Equitable & Supportive Care for effective PPH management, and this rely heavily on having a feasible and reliable method for blood-loss assessment.

OBS CYMRU Approach developed in Wales UK-4 pillar of PPH management:

1. Risk assessment—at time of antenatal visit and at time of admission in delivery unit
2. Early identification—blood loss to be calculated in each delivery
3. Multidisciplinary approach (MDT)—All including nursing staff, obstetrician or anesthetist should be involved in calculation of total blood loss.
4. ROTEM guided blood products managements
   Blood loss estimation remains a cornerstone for this approach.

METHODS OF BLOOD LOSS ESTIMATION

Visual Estimation

Visual estimation is the most commonly practiced method worldwide; however, it is highly subjective and imprecise. It consistently underestimates actual blood loss and contributes to delays in life-saving interventions. Tools such as Signaling a Postpartum Hemorrhage Emergency (SAPHE) mat, which is composed of superabsorbent polymer, nylon, pellon, and surgimat dressings. The mat is designed so that each square absorbs up to 50 mL of blood. Counting the number of blood-filled squares allows for an approximate calculation of the lost blood.

Moreover, it requires repeated timely training which has been seen to regress over time. Accuracy doesn't changes much with age, specialty and clinical experience.

Requires: Pictographs and repeat training for better results

Shortcomings: Being subjective there are 30–50% chances of underestimation in large blood losses

A systematic review and meta-analysis comparing diagnostic methods reported that quantitative techniques are significantly more accurate than visual estimation, although considerable heterogeneity exists across studies.

Quantitative Estimation

Quantitative estimation (QBL) involves measuring actual amount of blood loss. Associated with less chances of error (around 15%).

Gravimetric Method

The gravimetric technique involves weighing absorbent materials before and after use. FIGO recommends the formula:

$$(\text{Weight after} - \text{Weight before}) \div 1.05 = \text{Estimated blood volume}$$

where 1.05 g/mL represents the amount of blood lost. For the better understanding and memorizing 1 gm of weighted blood can be kept equal to 1 mL of blood loss.

Gravimetric methods are simple, inexpensive, and more accurate than visual estimation, though amniotic fluid contamination may reduce precision.

A 2018 Cochrane Review evaluating diagnostic accuracy reported that visual estimation has low sensitivity, whereas calibrated drapes combined with clinical observation demonstrated high sensitivity and specificity.

Volumetric Method

Volumetric measurement uses calibrated drapes, containers, or suction systems to quantify blood loss. While objective, workflow interruptions and mixed fluids (blood + amniotic fluid) may affect accuracy.

QBL combining both gravimetric and volumetric that is measuring blood loss using calibrated drapes, suction container, kidney trays containing liquid or clotted blood with weighing of soaked materials is currently the most reliable method. ACOG recommends quantitative techniques because they are substantially more accurate and improve early detection and timely response to PPH.

QBL should be team effort and requires interdisciplinary protocols made by multidisciplinary team. Process involves:

Vaginal Delivery

- Create dry weight list chart of delivery items that can get soaked
- Do first blood loss estimation after delivery of baby but before delivery of placenta. Record amount of fluid collected in calibrated drape
- Subtract preplacental fluid (liquor, urine and stools) from postplacental fluid (most likely blood). It is preferable to change underperineum calibrated drape (Dhaka/Dk drape) before delivery of placenta
- Weigh the wet delivery material and subtract their dry weight = 1 mL of blood loss
- Weigh all clots. Rule is 1 gm weight = 1 mL of blood loss
- Addition will give final blood loss.

Cesarean Delivery

- Label suction fluid after drainage of amniotic fluid
- Weigh the wet surgical drapes, mops for final blood loss quantification
- In case of placenta accreta spectrum low lithotomy with under perineum drapes can be applied.

Colorimetric and Image-based Techniques

Use of artificial intelligence technology, which uses colorimetric analysis and imaging software, can provide highly accurate blood-loss measurements, especially during cesarean deliveries, but these modalities are technologically demanding and costly, limiting routine use in low-resource settings. It requires further studies to validate these techniques.

Clinical Predictors and Physiological Indicators

Clinical markers help detect hemodynamic instability associated with blood loss.

- *Shock Index (SI):* SI > 0.9 indicates significant blood loss.
  A study by Pan et al. (2025) shows moderate diagnostic accuracy (sensitivity ~76%, specificity ~78%) for severe PPH.
- *Rule of 30:* A fall in systolic BP by 30 mm Hg, rise in HR by 30 bpm, or 30% drop in hematocrit suggests ~30% blood-volume loss.
- *Vital Signs:* Tachycardia and low systolic pressure are early markers of hypovolemia.
- *Urine output:* Reduced urine output reflects intravascular depletion.

Laboratory Parameters

Serial hemoglobin/hematocrit and coagulation profiles help in ongoing assessment but are limited during acute events due to delayed availability and it takes time to reflect the blood loss in blood parameters.

Imaging Techniques

Ultrasonographic assessment of IVC collapsibility or distensibility offers additional insight into intravascular volume status, though its use is limited in resource-constrained settings and requires training of individuals for the same.

Advances Technological Methods—Spectrophotometry

It allows the measurement of hemoglobin in the collected fluids and to make an accurate quantification of the actual blood volume (discounting other fluids such as amniotic fluid). It is quite accurate but high cost and availability in low-to medium-resource settings is an issue.

It is important to calculate cumulative blood loss in the first 24 h postpartum, not just immediately after birth. Hence it is essential to document soaked items and expelled clots, converting weights to volume and chart blood loss like urine output; intervene when thresholds are exceeded.

USEFUL STRATEGIES FOR IMPLEMENTATION OF QBL ESTIMATION

- Requires multidisciplinary training and adherence to established protocols
- Shift from subjective estimation to routine objective quantification
- Process maps guide implementation for vaginal and cesarean births
- Training and continuous updating of the team-Virtual Simulation training for PPH
- Enhancing team spirit and team response times
- Debriefing and risk management in every case of PPH
- Use of modified obstetric early warning scores in delivery units

Evidence on Improving Estimation Accuracy

Maslowitz et al. demonstrated through simulation-based training that team-based interval estimation improves accuracy compared to single-point estimation, though significant underestimation still persists.

An integrative review evaluating whether improved accuracy translates into better outcomes found limited evidence that enhanced blood-loss measurement alone reduces severe PPH or treatment delays. Tools and training improve measurement quality, but the downstream effect on maternal outcomes remains inconsistent.

Cumulative blood-loss assessment over the first 24 hours postpartum has greater clinical relevance than a single intrapartum estimate, as secondary PPH can occur after delivery.

The E-MOTIVE trial published in 2023 was a cluster-randomized study conducted in 80 secondary-level hospitals across LMICs, demonstrated that early, objective detection using calibrated drapes combined with immediate bundled first-line treatment significantly reduces severe PPH, maternal morbidity, and mortality.

KEY MESSAGE

- Quantification of blood loss is essential in all deliveries
- No single method provides a flawless approach to blood-loss estimation.
- Accuracy of QBL is dependent on proper technique and provider training.
- Combining quantitative methods with physiological indicators and robust clinical readiness aligned with FIGO's Obstetric care bundle approach is essential for reducing PPH-related morbidity and mortality.

SUGGESTED READING

1. American College of Obstetricians and Gynecologists (ACOG). Quantitative blood loss in obstetric hemorrhage. ACOG Committee Opinion No. 794. Obstet Gynecol. 2019;134:e150-6.
2. Bingham D, Jones R, et al. Cumulative blood loss measurement and the detection of postpartum hemorrhage. J Obstet Gynecol Neonatal Nurs. 2011.
3. Bose P, Regan F, Paterson-Brown S. Improving the accuracy of estimated blood loss at obstetric haemorrhage using clinical reconstructions. BJOG. 2006;113(8):919-24.
4. Diaz V, Abalos E, Carroli G. Methods for blood loss estimation after vaginal birth. Cochrane Database Syst Rev. 2018;9(9):CD010980.
5. Dipti A, Soucy Z, Surana A, et al. Inferior vena cava ultrasound to assess volume status in obstetric patients. J Ultrasound Med. 2012;31(7):1101-6.
6. Doctorvaladan SV, Jelks AT, Hsieh EW, Thurer RL, Zakowski MI, Lagrew DC. Accuracy of Blood Loss Measurement during Cesarean Delivery. AJP Rep. 2017;7(2):e93-e100.
7. FIGO Safe Motherhood Committee. FIGO postpartum haemorrhage guidelines: Prevention and treatment of postpartum haemorrhage. Int J Gynaecol Obstet. 2012;119(2):113-7.
8. Gallos ID, Papadopoulou A, Tsiami A, et al. Randomized trial of early detection and treatment of postpartum hemorrhage. N Engl J Med. 2023;389(12):1124-33.
9. Hancock A, Weeks AD, Lavender DT. Is accurate and reliable blood loss estimation the "crucial step" in early detection of postpartum haemorrhage: an integrative review of the literature. BMC Pregnancy Childbirth. 2015;15:230.
10. Hancock A, Weeks AD, Lavender T. Is accurate and reliable blood loss estimation the 'gold standard'? A systematic review. BJOG. 2015;122(5):618-27.
11. Lertbunnaphong T, Leetheeragul J, Manonai J, et al. Accuracy of the gravimetric method for estimation of postpartum blood loss: a systematic review. Arch Gynecol Obstet. 2016;294(5):1061-7.

12. Magann EF, Evans S, Hutchinson M, et al. Postpartum vital sign changes and early detection of hemorrhage. Am J Obstet Gynecol. 2005;193(3 Suppl):S45-7.
13. Makino Y, Miyake K, Okada A, Ikeda Y, Okada Y. Predictive accuracy of the shock index for severe postpartum hemorrhage in high-income countries: A systematic review and meta-analysis. J Obstet Gynaecol Res. 2022;48(8): 2027-37.
14. Maslovitz S, Barkai G, Lessing JB, et al. Improved accuracy for blood loss estimation in obstetric hemorrhage using simulation-based training. Obstet Gynecol. 2008;112(2 Pt 1):330–6.
15. Mohamed TAEH, Chandraharan E. Recognition and Management of Post-partum Hemorrhage. Matern Fetal Med. 2025;7(1):29-37.
16. O'Donnell C, Burns R. The 'rule of 30' in obstetric hemorrhage: clinical utility. Obstet Med. 2011;4(3):122-5.
17. Patel A, Goudar SS, Geller SE, et al. Drape estimation vs visual estimation of postpartum hemorrhage. Int J Gynaecol Obstet. 2006;93(3):220-4.
18. Say L, Chou D, Gemmill A, Tunçalp Ö, Moller AB, Daniels J, et al. Global causes of maternal death: a WHO systematic analysis. Lancet Glob Health. 2014;2(6):e323-33.
19. Shields LE, Goffman D, Caughey AB, et al. Laboratory markers in postpartum hemorrhage. Obstet Gynecol Clin North Am. 2020;47(2):409-24.
20. Stafford I, Dildy GA, Clark SL, et al. Visually estimated and calculated blood loss in vaginal and cesarean delivery. Obstet Gynecol. 2008;112(1):77-81.
21. Toledo P, McCarthy RJ, Burke CA, et al. The accuracy of blood loss estimation after simulated vaginal delivery. Anesth Analg. 2007;105(6):1736-40.

3 CHAPTER

Comparative Efficacy of Different Drugs in the Management of Postpartum Hemorrhage

Shashi L Kabra Maheshwari, Shalini V Singh

INTRODUCTION

Postpartum hemorrhage (PPH) is the leading direct cause of maternal mortality worldwide. If not timely managed, then the woman can die in 20–30 minutes. Aggressive management of PPH is the rule.

The first strategy is prevention, like correcting anemia and optimizing hemoglobin, active management of the third stage of labor (AMTSL) by giving an injection of Oxytocin 10 IU, within 1 minute of delivery. This prevents the incidence of PPH by approximately 50%. If the cold chain is not maintained or Oxytocin or is not available, then injection carbetocin 100 µg IM or IV or 600-µg Tab Misoprostol can be given for the prevention of PPH.

If PPH happens even after AMTSL, *uterine massage* and administration of Uterotonics are always the first line of management in treatment and prophylaxis. The triad of dilutional coagulopathy, hypo-fibrinogenemia, and hyperfibrinolysis develops rapidly in obstetric hemorrhage and timely correction of coagulopathy is essential to prevent progression to severe PPH, hysterectomy, multi organ dysfunction and death. Optimal use of these agents by understanding there efficacy, relative benefits and limitations in different clinical scenarios is key **(Table 1)**.

Among available hemostatic agents, *tranexamic acid (TXA), fibrinogen concentrates, or cryoprecipitate, and recombinant activated factor VII (rFVIIa)* target different segments of the hemostatic pathway. Early treatment of coagulopathy should be initiated alongside other management, in high-risk conditions, such as placental abruption or amniotic fluid embolism **(Flowcharts 1 and 2)**.

Coagulation factors are decreased due to physiological changes of pregnancy, therefore obstetric hemorrhage is unique as fibrinogen levels drop early and disproportionately **(Table 2)**. Hyperfibrinolysis sets in rapidly due to massive tissue plasminogen activator release. In massive hemorrhage, thrombin generation becomes inadequate. Therefore, three therapeutic questions arise:

1. Should fibrinolysis be inhibited? (TXA)
2. Should thrombin generation be pharmacologically boosted? (rFVIIa)
3. Should the clot substrate be replenished? (fibrinogen)

TABLE 1: Different uterotonics used for the initial management of PPH.

Drug	*Dose and route*	*Maximum dose*	*Precautions/Contraindications*	*Remarks*
Oxytocin	*IV (intravenous):* 20 units of oxytocin diluted in 1 L of fluid at a rate of 40 drops per minute	*IV fluids with oxytocin:* Do not exceed 3 liters of IV fluids containing oxytocin in total	Do not administer as an IV bolus	Drug of choice both for prophylaxis and treatment
Carbetocin	100 µg IM (Intramuscular) or IV	100 µg	*Contraindications:* Avoid use in women with cardiovascular disorders, hepatic or renal disease, epilepsy, or known drug hypersensitivity/sensitivity	Used only for prophylaxis of PPH
Ergometrine/ Methyler-gometrine	IM or IV: 0.2 mg. Repeat every 15 minutes	Up to 5 doses (total 1.0 mg)	*Contraindications: Avoid use in patients with* hypertension, pre-eclampsia/eclampsia, cardiac disease, or retained placenta	Not used for prophylaxis of PPH
15-methyl Prostaglandin F2α (carboprost)	IM: *Administer* 0.25 mg *intramuscularly*; repeat every 15 minutes if required, *based on clinical response*	Up to 8 doses (Total 2 mg)	*Contraindications:* Avoid carboprost in patients with asthma, cardiovascular, renal, or hepatic disease, hypotension, pulmonary edema, uterine infection, or a history of known hypersensitivity Do not administer intravenously (IV)	Not used for prophylaxis
Misoprostol (PGE1)	Sublingual: *Administer* 800 µg *sublingually*	Not more than 1,600 µg (Total)	Use with caution in patients with cardiovascular disease; may cause fever or chills	Can not be used for treatment if already used for prophylaxis

Note: The total dose of methylergonovine is 5 doses that is 1 g, and the total dose of carboprost is 8 doses that is 2 g, but the repeat dose is not to be given if the patient does not respond to one dose. Then we *should escalate to the next uterotonic in line*.

Flowchart 1: Practical Algorithm of PPH bundle.

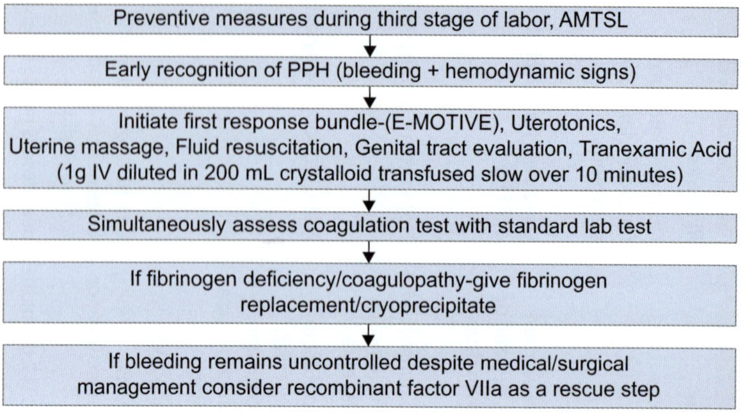

Flowchart 2: Hemostatic pathways and point of action of different drugs (green box).

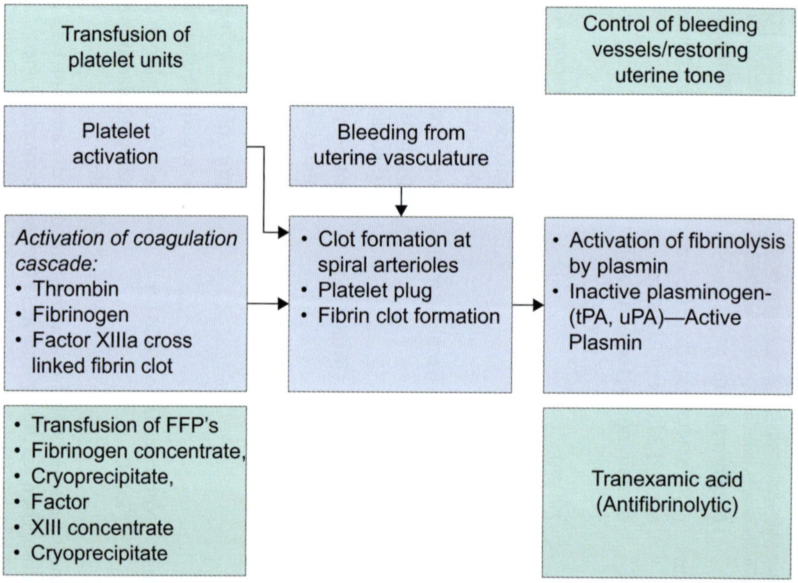

What is 'best'? Depends on the context of clinical Scenario? (Evidence based)

- For *prevention of PPH* (active management of third stage/prophylaxis), the most effective regimens (in RCT data) appear to be the combinations *ergometrine + oxytocin, carbetocin,* or *misoprostol + oxytocin* — all superior to oxytocin alone.
- *Carbetocin may offer the best balance of efficacy and side-effect profile* but evidence is limited.
- For *active PPH treatment,* especially if uterotonics alone are insufficient, or bleeding partly due to trauma/coagulopathy—*TXA* is increasingly

TABLE 2: Comparison of Hemostatic agents.

	Tranexamic acid (TXA)	*Fibrinogen concentrate/ cryoprecipitate*	*Recombinant factor VIIA (rFVII-A)*
Mechanism of action	Antifibrinolytic drug Synthetic lysine analoge that blocks lysine-binding sites on plasminogen, preventing plasmin formation and its binding to fibrin. This prevents fibrin degradation and reduces clot breakdown, helping to maintain clot stability and control bleeding	• Earliest and most critical coagulation factor in coagulation pathway • Levels *<200 mg/dL* strongly predict progression to severe PPH • Maintaining fibrinogen above *300–400 mg/dL* improves hemostasis • Replaces clot substrate	Activates the extrinsic pathway by binding to tissue factor and activating factors IX and X, boosting thrombin generation and formation of stable clots
Evidence	• *The WOMAN Trial* (*n* = 20,060) showed a *31% reduction in death due to bleeding* when TXA was given within 3 hours of birth • *TXA also* significantly decreased the need for laparotomy, *with* no observed increase in thromboembolic events	*OBS2, the FIDEL and European trauma databases* support early fibrinogen replacement to reduce transfusion requirements	Observational studies (e.g., Shahi et al.) showed significant reduction in blood loss
Clinical efficacy	• Most Effective when administered *early*, particularly in cases of traumatic PPH or where there is evidence of hyperfibrinolysis • It reduces ongoing blood loss but does not correct low fibrinogen or poor clot quality	*Most Effective when PPH is accompanied by:* massive hemorrhage, hypo-fibrinogenemia, Dilutional coagulopathy, Amniotic fluid embolism, DIC	• *Most effective in:* Refractory PPH unresponsive to medical/ surgical management • Persistent bleeding even after caesarean hysterectomy, cases with adequate • Fibrinogen levels

Contd…

Contd…

	Tranexamic acid (TXA)	*Fibrinogen concentrate/ cryoprecipitate*	*Recombinant factor VIIA (rFVII-A)*
Dose	1g IV over 10 minutes; second dose 1 g after 30 minutes if bleeding persists	• *Fibrinogen concentrate:* 2–4 g initially • *Cryoprecipitate:* 3–4 pools (approx. 6–8 g fibrinogen)	90 µg/kg; second dose may be given if bleeding continues
Advantages	• Rapid onset • Safe, inexpensive • Proven mortality benefit • Easy storage, administration • Useful across all types of PPH	• Directly restores fibrin substrate • Rapid improves fibrinogen level • Essential in DIC and consumptive coagulopathy	• Rapid hemostatic effect in selected cases • Useful in near-miss situations
Limitations	• Ineffective in severe hypofibrinogenemia • Does not replace clotting factors	• Cryoprecipitate requires thawing and cross-matching • Ineffective without controlling fibrinolysis or thrombin generation	• Works poorly when fibrinogen <150 mg/dL • Costly • Thromboembolic risk (venous or arterial) • Not a substitute for conventional transfusion

TABLE 3: Efficacy and safety of different drugs.

Efficacy	*Safety*
• Most Effective first line-*oxytocin* • Refractory Atony-Ergometrine, carboprost are superior but has side effects • *TXA* enhances survival but only an adjunct	• Safest uterotonics: *Oxytocin* • Max Side effects and contraindications: *Ergometrine, carboprost*

standard as an adjunct, with proven mortality benefit (when given early) and generally acceptable safety.

- When comparing Misoprostol vs Oxytocin directly (for prevention), the most recent participants-data meta-analysis (2024) found *no advantage* of misoprostol—possibly even a higher risk of PPH ≥500 mL or severe PPH—compared to oxytocin.
- Among all comparison on lines of prevention of maternal mortality no difference has been yet suggested over different drugs **(Table 3)**.

TABLE 4: Strengthening PPH care pathways.

TXA first-line	*Fibrinogen factor-targeted*	*r-FVIIa*
Hemostatic agent- affordable, easy storage, no laboratory test needed	• Expensive, often unavailable, requires coagulation assays • Targeted when severe PPH, Blood loss >1,000 mL with clinical signs of coagulopathy, bleeding refractory to utertonics/TXA	• Restricted to life saving option- High cost/low availability, risk of thrombosis • In scenarios of persistent PPH despite all medical and surgical measures, and coagulation factor supplementation done to best way possible

ADAPTATION OVER USE IN LOW RESOURCE SETTINGS

Low resource settings have challenges of limited blood-bank capacity, lack of 24-hour laboratory support, delays in transport and referral, shortages of skilled providers, and restricted access to advanced hemostatic agents. Following operational adaptations along with *strengthening PPH care pathways* should be employed **(Table 4)**.

TAKE HOMF MESSAGE

- Oxytocin is the preferred first-line therapy, while misoprostol, methylergometrine, Carboprost, and tranexamic acid serve valuable roles in specific clinical contexts or in refractory cases.
- TXA is the only agent with proven mortality benefit.
- Fibrinogen is the earliest coagulation factor to fall, and hypo-fibrinogenaemia <200 mg/dL predicts worsening haemorrhage. Fibrinogen replacement either with fibrinogen concentrate or cryoprecipitate is therefore essential in moderate to severe bleeding or when DIC is evolving.
- r-FVIIa is a potent but last-resort therapy for refractory haemorrhage when other measures fail. Its use requires adequate fibrinogen, platelets, pH, and temperature.
- Used in a stepwise escalation, these agents significantly reduce maternal morbidity and mortality in PPH.

SUGGESTED READING

1. Bohren MA, Miller S, Mammoliti KM, Galadanci H, Fawcus S, Moran N, et al. Early detection and a treatment bundle strategy for postpartum haemorrhage: a mixed-methods process evaluation. Lancet Glob Health. 2025;13(2):e329-44.
2. Collins PW, Cannings-John R, Bruynseels D, Mallaiah S, Dick J, Elton C, et al. Viscoelastometric-guided early fibrinogen concentrate replacement during postpartum haemorrhage: OBS2, a double-blind randomized controlled trial. Br J Anaesth. 2017;119(3):411-21.
3. Conwell J, Katz D. Haemostatic agents in the management of obstetric haemorrhage. BJA Educ. 2024;24(11):426-32.
4. Ducloy-Bouthors AS, Mercier FJ, Grouin JM, Bayoumeu F, Corouge J, Le Gouez A, et al., FIDEL working group. Early and systematic administration of

fibrinogen concentrate in postpartum haemorrhage following vaginal delivery: the FIDEL randomised controlled trial. BJOG. 2021;128(11):1814-23.

5. Escobar MF, Nassar AH, Theron G, Barnea ER, Nicholson W, Ramasauskaite D, et al., FIGO Safe Motherhood and Newborn Health Committee. FIGO recommendations on the management of postpartum hemorrhage 2022. Int J Gynaecol Obstet. 2022;157 Suppl 1(Suppl 1):3-50.
6. Evidence reviews for pharmacological management of postpartum haemorrhage: Intrapartum care: Evidence review O. London: National Institute for Health and Care Excellence (NICE); 2023.
7. Flanagan M, Au N, Patabendige M, Rattan A, Samanta R, Sahota D, et al. Misoprostol Versus Oxytocin for the Prevention of Postpartum Haemorrhage: A Systematic Review and Meta-Analysis Including Individual Participant Data. BJOG. 2025;132(10):1364-77.
8. Gallos I, Devall A, Martin J, Middleton L, Beeson L, Galadanci H, et al. Randomized trial of early detection and treatment of postpartum haemorrhage. N Engl J Med. 2023;389(1):11-21.
9. Gallos ID, Papadopoulou A, Man R, Athanasopoulos N, Tobias A, Price MJ, et al. Uterotonic agents for preventing postpartum haemorrhage: a network meta-analysis. Cochrane Database Syst Rev. 2018;12(12):CD011689.
10. Gallos ID, Williams HM, Price MJ, Merriel A, Gee H, Lissauer D, et al. Uterotonic agents for preventing postpartum haemorrhage: a network meta-analysis. Cochrane Database Syst Rev. 2025;4(4):CD011689.
11. Ker K, Sentilhes L, Shakur-Still H, Madar H, Deneux-Tharaux C, Saade G, et al. Tranexamic acid for postpartum bleeding: a systematic review and individual patient data meta-analysis of randomised controlled trial. Lancet. 2024;404(10463):1657-67.
12. Magon N, Babu K. Recombinant Factor VIIa in Post-partum Hemorrhage: A New Weapon in Obstetrician's Armamentarium. N Am J Med Sci. 2012; 4(4):157-62.
13. Mengoli C, Franchini M, Marano G, Pupella S, Vaglio S, Marietta M, et al. The use of fibrinogen concentrate for the management of trauma-related bleeding: a systematic review and meta-analysis. Blood Transfus. 2017;15(4): 318-24.
14. PW Collins, Whyte CS, de Lloyd L, Narwal A, Bell SF, Gill N, et al. Acute obstetric coagulopathy is associated with excess plasmin generation and proteolysis of fibrinogen and factor V. Blood Adv. 2025;9(11):2751-62.
15. Royal College of Obstetricians and Gynaecologists. (2025). Prevention and Management of Postpartum Haemorrhage (Green-top Guideline No. 52). [online] Available from https://www.rcog.org.uk/guidance/browse-all-guidance/green-top-guidelines/prevention-and-management-of-postpartum-haemorrhage-green-top-guideline-no-52/ [Last accessed December, 2025].
16. Sahin AS, Ozkan S. Treatment of Obstetric Hemorrhage with Fibrinogen Concentrate. Med Sci Monit. 2019;25:1814-21.
17. Shahi P, Pritam A, Sinha A, Pratima, Sinha G, Bibha K, et al. Early intervention with recombinant factor VIIa in severe postpartum hemorrhage: a retrospective observational study for evaluation of safety and efficacy of recombinant activated factor VII. Int J Reprod, Contracep, Obstetr Gynecol. 2025;14(8): 2504-9.

18. WHO. (2025). Consolidated guidelines for the prevention, diagnosis and treatment of postpartum haemorrhage. [online] Available from https://www.who.int/publications/i/item/9789240115637 [Last accessed December, 2025].
19. WOMAN Trial Collaborators. Effect of early tranexamic acid administration on mortality, hysterectomy, and other morbidities in women with post-partum haemorrhage (WOMAN): an international, randomised, double-blind, placebo-controlled trial. Lancet. 2017;389(10084):2105-16.
20. World Health Organization. WHO recommendations on the assessment of postpartum haemorrhage and use of a treatment bundle. Geneva; WHO; 2023.

4 CHAPTER

Principles of Monitoring and Communication in Management of Postpartum Hemorrhage

Suchitra N Pandit, Ami Surti

INTRODUCTION

Postpartum hemorrhage (PPH) is an obstetric emergency that requires a coordinated multidisciplinary approach which involves good communication including an obstetrician, perinatologist, anesthesiologist, hematologist, blood bank, interventional radiologist and skilled nursing staff for accurate assessment of blood loss, monitoring of maternal signs and symptoms, fluid, blood and blood product replacement, and arrest of the source of the hemorrhage. Analysis of healthcare team performances for women who suffered a PPH, showed that focusing on team relationships and culture are critical influences on teamwork behaviors and outcomes.

Effective monitoring in managing PPH needs an accurate blood loss assessment using quantitative techniques and continuous monitoring of vital signs to detect early signs of hypovolemic shock. Clear communication is essential, utilizing teamwork with defined roles, closed-loop communication strategies, and maintaining situational awareness among multidisciplinary teams to ensure a coordinated and rapid response.

PRINCIPLES OF MONITORING

Early detection of PPH and the continuous assessment of the patient's condition is the first step for effective monitoring.

Quantitative Blood Loss Assessment

Visual estimation of blood loss is often inaccurate. Quantitative blood loss (QBL) methods, such as weighing blood-soaked materials and using calibrated collection drapes/canisters, are recommended for a more accurate assessment and to avoid delayed intervention.

Measuring blood loss as accurately as possible is essential for identifying the severity of hemorrhage and assessing patient's response to hemorrhage. According to a pictorial reference guide to aid visual estimation of blood loss, the amount of blood estimations are soiled sanitary towel (30 mL), soaked sanitary towel (100 mL), small soaked swab 10 × 10 (60 mL), large soaked swab 45 × 45 (350 mL), and full kidney dish (500 mL). Also, blood in aspiratory tubes (includes amnion fluid as well) under buttocks drapes and surgery site (blood pooling) needs to be considered. But, in visual estimations, rate of misdiagnosis is around 35–50%. Therefore, instead of estimated blood loss (EBL), since it is always very difficult as well as late, quantitative measurement is recommended. The following equation is used when calculating blood loss of a blood-soaked item:

WET item gram weight – DRY item weight = Milliliters of blood within the item

If there is a birth with no rupture of the amniotic sac, the following volumes can be used to estimate the contribution of amniotic fluid in the aspiratory tubes; at term, it is approximately 700 mL, where it could be 300 mL or 1400 mL in oligohydramnios and polyhydramnios, respectively, as indicated.

Continuous Vital Sign Monitoring

Vital signs should be frequently and regularly assessed (e.g., every 5–15 minutes, depending on severity).

Key indicators are:

- Heart rate (tachycardia can be an early sign)
- Blood pressure (hypotension is a later, more severe sign)
- Respiratory rate
- Oxygen saturation
- Temperature
- Conscious state

- *Assessment of uterine tone and involution:* The uterus should be regularly palpated to assess its tone. A soft, "boggy" uterus indicates atony, the most common cause of PPH, requiring immediate massage and uterotonic medications.
- *Monitoring of urine output:* An indwelling urinary catheter should be inserted to monitor urine output, which is a key indicator of renal perfusion and overall hemodynamic stability.
- *Laboratory investigations:* Serial blood tests, including complete blood count (hemoglobin and hematocrit levels), coagulation profile (fibrinogen, platelets), and blood gases (lactate), help guide resuscitation and identify coagulopathies.
- *Fluid balance charting:* An accurate record of all input (IV fluids, blood products) and output (urine, blood loss) is essential for fluid management. During bleeding, replacement of extracellular fluid losses with isotonic crystalloids in a timely protocol-based manner is suggested. Infusion of colloids provides hemodynamic stabilization with less tissue oedema when compared with crystalloids.

Dilutional coagulopathy can be worsened with aggressive volume loading in severe bleeding. So, restrictive volume replacement (1–2 mL crystalloid for each 1 mL blood loss) to avoid secondary hypervolemia and dilution of coagulation factors that would further aggravate coagulopathy are of utmost importance. Maintaining normovolemia is crucial to compensate for the losses and provide hemodynamic stabilization in this patient population.

PRINCIPLES OF COMMUNICATION

Clear, timely, and interprofessional communication is critical for effective teamwork and a coordinated response, especially in an emergency setting.

- *Early activation of emergency protocols:* Healthcare providers must know and promptly use local escalation procedures (e.g., PPH Alert/Coded calls) to involve senior clinical assistance and the multidisciplinary team (midwives, obstetricians, anesthetists, lab personnel, blood bank).
- *Clear role allocation and leadership:* During an emergency, a clear leader should be identified to coordinate the response and delegate specific roles and tasks (e.g., assessing blood loss, administering medications, documenting events) to ensure all necessary actions are covered and avoid confusion.
- *Closed-loop communication:* Messages must be clearly formulated, delivered, heard, and understood, often confirmed back by the receiver (closed-loop) to prevent miscommunication and errors.
- *SBAR (situation, background, assessment, recommendation) was originally developed in the military context to create a reliable consistent process to facilitate concise, clear, focused communication. SBAR* is a communication tool used in PPH to provide a structured, concise, and clear report of the patient's condition to other healthcare providers. It helps ensure consistent and effective communication during a critical event by outlining the current situation, relevant history, healthcare professional's evaluation, and what action is needed. When transferring care or escalating to a different team or facility, a structured handover process ensures all critical information is conveyed accurately.
- *Situation:* State the patient's current status and description of the immediate problem.

  Example for PPH: "The patient is bleeding heavily from the genital tract and her heart rate is increasing."
- *Background:*
  - *Provide relevant context:* Include details like the patient's diagnosis, recent procedures, and history.
  - *Example for PPH:* "She delivered vaginally two hours ago, and her placenta was delivered intact. There's no history of clotting disorders."

- *Assessment:*
  - Share your professional evaluation based on the situation and background, what do you think is happening?
  - *Example for PPH:* "I believe this is a case of uterine atony due to the heavy bleeding. She also has some trauma to the genital tract."
- *Recommendation:*
  - State clearly what you need or what needs to happen next: Be specific about what you want from the person you are communicating with.
  - *Example for PPH:* "I need you to come to the room to assess the patient. I need someone to call for a PPH trolley and keep two units of blood ready."
- *Diligent documentation:* A designated team member (scribe) should record events systematically, including vital signs, assessments, medications, fluid/blood products given, and the patient's response to management. This is vital for continuity of care and later review.
- *Patient and family communication:* It is very essential as they must be told about what is happening, why it is happening, and how it is being managed. Postpartum debriefing after the event is also recommended to discuss the experience and any future concerns.
- *Team debriefing and simulation training:* Regular multidisciplinary team training (Drills) and post-event debriefings are essential to practice skills, identify system issues, improve relational factors (trust, respect, shared knowledge), and improve future performance.
- Drills in PPH are simulated emergency response exercises for health-care teams to improve their readiness, coordination, and effectiveness in managing severe bleeding after childbirth. These drills, often using robotic simulators, help staff practice key skills like accurately estimating blood loss, using medical interventions such as uterine massage or tampons, and communicating effectively under pressure. Studies show that these simulations can lead to better patient outcomes, including a significant reduction in the likelihood of complications like hysterectomy, ICU admission, and maternal death.

CONCLUSION

Postpartum hemorrhage (PPH) is an obstetric emergency that requires effective teamwork under complex conditions.

Effective monitoring techniques and clarity in communication amongst the health care team is crucial to improving outcomes. Regular drills and use of simulators help the team to work together in a efficient and coordinated manner. Clear communication is essential, utilizing teamwork with defined roles, closed-loop communication strategies, and maintaining situational awareness among multidisciplinary teams to ensure a coordinated and rapid response.

KEY MESSAGES

- Postpartum hemorrhage (PPH) is an obstetric emergency that requires effective teamwork under complex conditions.
- Principles of monitoring and communication are crucial for the effective, multidisciplinary management of PPH.
- Effective monitoring in managing PPH needs an accurate blood loss assessment using quantitative techniques and continuous monitoring of vital signs to detect early signs of hypovolemic shock.
- *SBAR* is a communication tool used in PPH to provide a structured, concise, and clear report of the patient's condition to other healthcare providers. It helps ensure consistent and effective communication during a critical event by outlining the current situation, relevant history, healthcare professional's evaluation, and what action is needed. When transferring care or escalating to a different team or facility, a structured handover process ensures all critical information is conveyed accurately
- Regular drills and use of simulators help the team to work together in a efficient and coordinated manner.

SUGGESTED READING

1. Bose P, Regan F, Paterson-Brown S. Improving the accuracy of estimated blood loss at obstetric hemorrhage using clinical reconstructions. BJOG. 2006;113(8):919-24.
2. Brace RA, Wolf EJ. Normal amniotic fluid volume changes throughout pregnancy. Am J Obstet Gynecol. 1989;161(2):382-8.
3. Irawati R, Widodo A, Yulian V. The Effective Communication using SBAR (Situation, Background, Assessment, Recommendation) of Patient Handover in Inpatient Installation. Jurnal Berita IImu Keperawatan. 2025;18(1):47-55.
4. Kozek-Langenecker SA, Ahmed AB, Afshari A, Albaladejo P, Aldecoa C, Barauskas G, et al. Management of severe perioperative bleeding guidelines from the European Society of Anaesthesiology: first update 2016. Eur J Anaesthesiol. 2017;34(6):332-95.
5. Mendez-Figueroa H, Bell CS, Wagner SM, Pedroza C, Gupta M, Mulder I, et al. Postpartum hemorrhage drills or simulations and adverse outcomes: a systematic review and Bayesian meta-analysis. J Matern Fetal Neonatal Med. 2022;35(26):10416-27.
6. Muñoz M, Stensballe J, Ducloy-Bouthors AS, Bonnet MP, De Robertis E, Fornet I, et al. Patient blood management in obstetrics: prevention and treatment of postpartum haemorrhage. A nata consensus statement. Blood Transfus. 2019;17(2):112-36.

5 CHAPTER

The Success Story of SR Cannula

Samartha Ram H, Sruthi AV

INTRODUCTION

The WHO's latest report estimates that approximately *2.6 lakh maternal deaths* occurred globally in the year 2023. Almost 20 per cent of deaths (56,000) occurred in India. In developing countries, postpartum hemorrhage (PPH) remains the leading cause amounting to 50%, and atonic PPH is the cause in 29.6% of cases. Majority of these deaths occurred in peripheral centers with sub-optimal facilities. Even though some risk factors like obstructed prolonged labor, accidental hemorrhage, and big babies are known to cause atonic PPH, it is not very clear why some women develop atonic PPH and why some women do not. For the same reason this problem cannot be predictable. The only management strategy even today is 'watchful expectancy,' and act immediately when the problem arises. Simpler techniques like uterine massage, uterotonics drugs, uterine packing, and balloon tamponade can be practiced in low resource settings. Techniques like B-Lynch suturing, stepwise de-vascularization, internal iliac ligation, and uterine artery embolization are available only at higher medical centers. These higher techniques are not within the reach of every parturient woman when simpler techniques fail.

In low resource settings, unpredictable sudden massive bleeding makes it difficult to organize competent manpower, compatible blood and transport to higher medical centers. Many times, mothers die on roads while being transported to higher medical centers due to hypovolemic shock. In some women, the speed with which the hemorrhage kills the mother is so rapid, that the usually quoted first 1 or 2 hours as "Golden hours" is missing. Sometimes, the women succumb to death just within 1–1.5 hours after the onset of bleeding. The rapidity with which some women slip in to coagulation failure and multiorgan dysfunction syndrome from hemorrhagic shock is alarming. Because of these complex reasons, the maternal mortality is not coming down in low resource settings. There is every need for a simpler and sure technique which can stop bleeding, or at least stop bleeding temporarily to buy some time to tide over the crisis.

CONCEPT BEHIND SUCTION TAMPONADE WITH SR PPH SUCTION CANNULA

Creating negative pressure inside the uterine cavity with a specially designed uterine cannula *(SR PPH Cannula)*, results in shrinking of uterus which can assist the natural physiological process of contraction and retraction to stop atonic bleeding **(Fig. 1)**.

How Negative Pressure Works?

When negative pressure applied, the soft cervical tissues get sucked in to the perforations of cervical portion of the cannula and become adherent. The uterus becomes a closed cavity. Further continuation of negative pressure results in constriction, contraction, and firm retraction of uterus on the surface of cannula to stop atonic bleeding **(Fig. 1)**. This process assists the natural physiological mechanism of contraction and retraction.

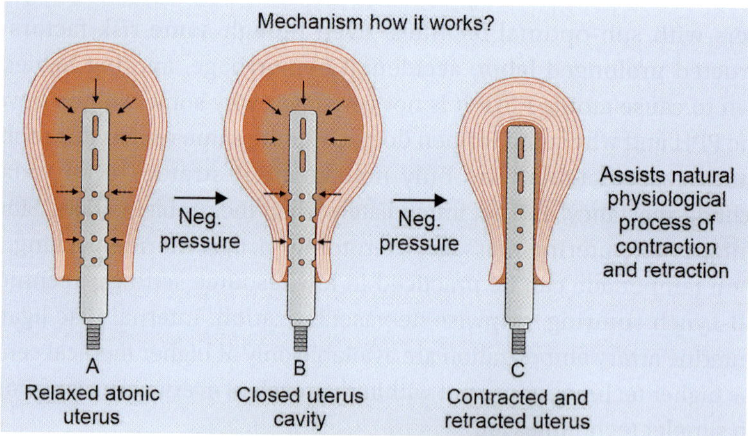

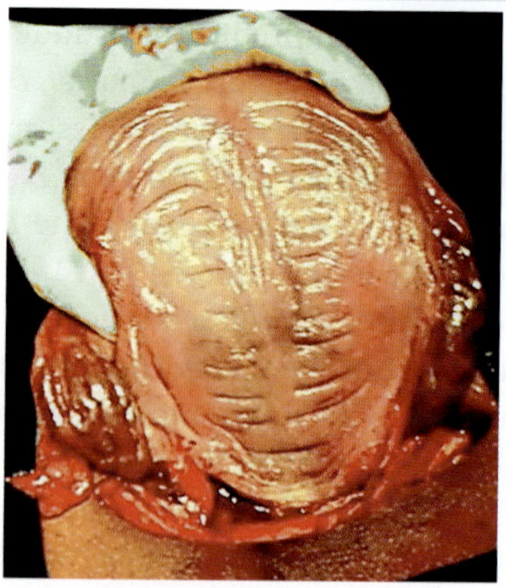

Fig. 1: Mechanisms how negative pressure inside the uterine cavity stops atonic bleeding.

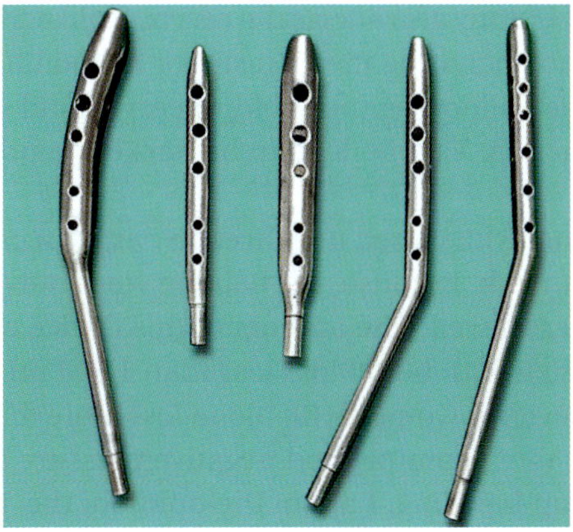

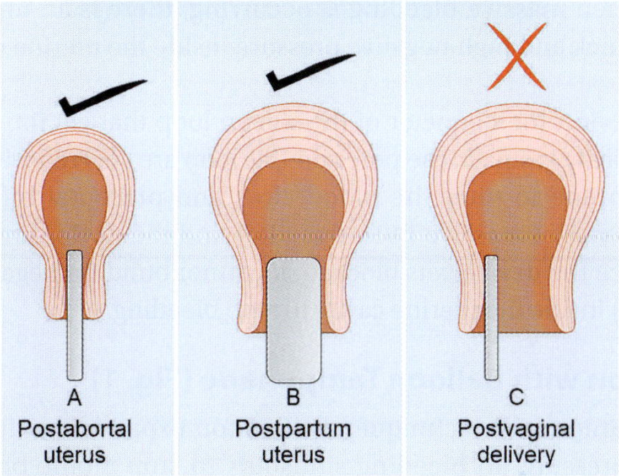

Fig. 2: Different sizes of cannulas to match different cervical dilatations and different uterocervical lengths. Postabortion uterus needs thin cannula (A). Immediate postpartum uterus needs larger diameter cannula (B). Thin cannula cannot achieve closed uterine cavity in immediate postpartum uterus (C).

Achieving effective negative pressure of 650 mm inside the uterine cavity is the fundamental requirement to achieve suction tamponade effect. This is possible only when we achieve a closed uterine cavity. Different obstetric bleeding situations have different cervical dilatations and different utero-cervical lengths. It is not possible to achieve close uterine cavity with a single design cannula. We need different diameter cannulas with different hole indicis to stop bleeding **(Fig. 2)**.

Comparison with Impress Suction Tamponade Device (Jada System)

In this device, E D Altton et al. provided fluid inflatable balloon to plug the cervix. When 4–5 cm of cervical dilatation is present, this balloon can effectively plug the cervix to achieve the closed uterine cavity. In cases of massive atonic PPH, atony also affects the cervix. Unlike with SR PPH suction cannula, there is no anchoring mechanism for balloon to anchor to cervix. In such a case, this balloon cannot hold to cervix, and get expelled when the uterus starts acting. Vagina need to be packed to prevent this balloon expulsion.

When PPH occur, with closed uneffaced cervix as in cases of elective CS, this device cannot work. Because, the balloon stays outside the cervix and cannot plug the cervix well. The authors of this device recommend to use this device in women with blood loss less than 1,500 mL. But SR Cannula, can stop bleeding even in women with blood loss more than 1,500 mL.

In this system, the recommended negative pressure is 70 to 90 mm Hg for one hour to stop bleeding. I am of the opinion; this is a week negative pressure. When massive bleeding is occurring, there is an urgent need to build up a quick and high negative pressure inside the uterine cavity to stop bleeding.

In this device, the diameter of the silicon loop that get introduced in to the uterine cavity is small. The pores on this loop are covered with something like a membrane to filter the blood clots and placental bits to prevent clogging. In case of massive PPH, this filter and the device are likely to get blocked. Once the device gets blocked, it cannot build up negative pressure (tamponade) inside the uterine cavity to stop bleeding.

Comparison with Balloon Tamponade (Fig. 1)

In balloon tamponade technique, the balloon expands the uterine cavity, and exerts pressure on bleeding sinusoids to stop atonic bleeding. This method works against the principle of physiological contraction and retraction of uterus.

Some amount of muscle tone must be present in uterine muscle for the balloon system to work (Tamponade test). With complete uterine atony, balloon tamponade cannot work. Suction tamponade system works even when complete atony of uterus is present. We need at least 20 to 30 minutes time to organize balloon system. If cannula system is organized before the delivery of the baby, hardly it takes less than a minute tine for insertion of cannula and application of negative pressure. The bleeding stops just within 2–3 minutes of time.

DESCRIPTION OF UTERINE VACUUM RETRACTION SYSTEM

- *SR PPH suction cannulas:* Five different sizes of cannulas are made to match different cervical dilatations and for different uterocervical lengths **(Fig. 2)**.
- Perforations on fundal portion of the cannula are large and round (6 mm), and on cervical portion they are round and small (5 mm).

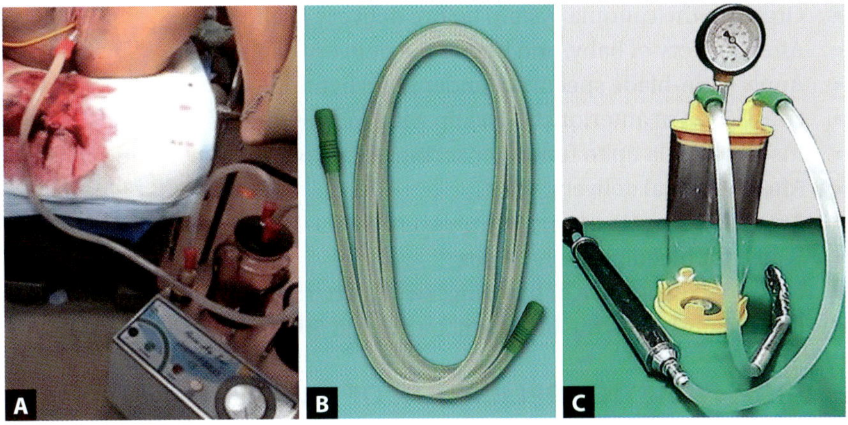

Figs. 3A to C: Cannula inserted into the uterine cavity and connected to high vacuum suction machine (A). Thick walled not easily collapsible flexible plastic suction tube (B). Manual suction pump, equally effective to create negative pressure inside the uterine cavity (C).

- Vaginal portion of the cannula do not have any holes **(Fig. 2)**.
- Thin long cannula is also used as a suction tube introducer while applying cannula during cesarean section.
- *High vacuum suction machine* or vacuum suction pump, which can produce a negative pressure up to 650mm within 1mnt **(Fig. 3A)**.
- Thick walled not easily collapsible flexible plastic suction tube **(Fig. 3B)** (Disposable suction tubes available in market can be used)

APPLICATION SR CANNULA FOR ATONIC PPH DURING VAGINAL DELIVERY

- Connect cannula nipple to one end of suction tube
- The other end of suction tube should be connected to suction machine
- Apply wide-blade speculum under good lighting
- Grasp 5 cm of anterior cervical lip with sponge forceps
- Insert cannula up to fundus ensuring all perforations lie inside cervix
- Apply 650 mm Hg negative pressure for 10–15 minutes
- Repeat every hour for 2 more sessions.
- Start oxytocin infusion simultaneously
- Bleeding stops within ~2 minutes

PROPHYLACTIC APPLICATION DURING VAGINAL DELIVERY

Prophylactic application of SR Cannula is done for women who are at risk of developing atonic PPH like anemia complicating pregnancy, PIH, placental abruption, hydramnios, and multifetal pregnancy.

- Organize the cannula system before delivery itself
- After delivery of baby, and before the delivery of placenta
- Apply wide-blade speculum under good lighting
- Grasp 5 cm of anterior cervical lip with sponge forceps
- Insert cannula up to fundus ensuring all perforations lie inside cervix.
- After placental delivery,
- Apply 650 mm Hg of negative pressure for 10–15 minutes
- Watch for bleeding for 1–2 hour
- In case of recurrence of bleeding, switch on the suction machine
- Blood collected in the bottle will be around 50–100 mL.

PROPHYLACTIC APPLICATION OF SR CANNULA DURING CAESAREAN DELIVERY

- After placental delivery, assess cervical dilatation with index finger
- Fix the appropriate size of cannula to one end of suction tube.
- The other end should be fixed to suction tube introducer
- Pass introducer through uterine incision → cervix → vagina
- Assistant retrieves it vaginally, and connects to the suction machine
- Ensure cervical portion of the cannula in cervical region.
- Keep the cut edges of the wound together, and then apply negative pressure.
- Close uterine incision while suction is on

When to Remove Cannula?

- In case of prophylactic application, cannula can be removed after 1–2 hours
- In case of frank atonic PPH, cannula can be removed after 8–12 hours
- After massive PPH, cannula can be removed after 24 hours
- After removal of cannula, if bleeding recurs, cannula should be reapplied.

How to Remove Cannula?

- Vaginally, push 10 mL of 5% xylocaine jelly around cervix.
- After 10 minutes, apply gentle traction on suction tube and cannula with left hand.
- Right index finger should be inserted between the cannula and cervix
- Gently release the stuck cervical tissues from the holes of cervical cannula
- Cannula comes out easily.

Results from Our Studies

- Complete cessation of bleeding in all cases within 4 minutes
- Blood collected in suction bottle ranged from 100–200 mL

- Significantly reduced the need for blood transfusion, laparotomy, and other major surgeries.
- Effective even in cases of coagulation failure[5]

SPECIAL APPLICATIONS

Bleeding after MTP, Vesicular Mole Extraction, and Secondary PPH

- Long slender cannula is developed for this purpose.
- Stops bleeding reliably.
- We are coming out with another cannula for cervical and scar ectopic pregnancies.

Coagulation Failure and DIC

Reported success in tertiary care centers including Calicut, Thrissur, Tirupati, Hubli and Jaipur.

Transporting Women with PPH

- Manual suction pump is used for this purpose **(Fig. 3C)**.
- Equally effective, and works without power.

ON GOING RESEARCH

SR PPH Suction Cannula to be Added to Active Management of Third Stage of Labor

In spite of regularly using active management of third stage of labor (AMTSL) in every labor, atonic PPH deaths are occurring continuously. In peripheral centers with suboptimal facilities, we recommend application of SR Cannula to all women after placental delivery, both in cases of vaginal and Caesarean deliveries. This minimizes blood loss, avoids the need for blood transfusion, and helps for an excellent postnatal recovery. Also, we are coming out with another cannula for managing cervical and scar ectopic pregnancies.

Who are all Required to be Trained?

- Obstetricians
- MBBS doctors
- AYUSH practitioners
- Staff nurses
- ANMs

  Universal training is recommended to reduce maternal mortality.

FIELD EXPERIENCES OF SR CANNULA

Handson Training Program at SVMC Tirupati, 6 Months Report

- 6,446 deliveries
- 34 refractory PPH cases treated
- Bleeding stopped in 100% cases
- Zero major surgeries
- Received Certificate of Excellence at AP Health Festival

Pilot Study on SR Cannula and Oral Hydration Therapy (OHT) at Chittoor District of AP

- 8,396 deliveries during the first 3 months **(Table 1)**
- SR Cannula used in 1,503 cases
- Zero maternal deaths due to PPH
- Major reduction in need for blood transfusion.
- Long-term MMR (5 years performance) in the district, brought down to ~33.3 **(Table 2)**

Another very significant observation, 16 Preeclampsia related deaths occurred during 2017–18, whereas only one death occurred during 2022–23. This clearly shows the efficacy of OHT in preventing preeclampsia related deaths. *Oral Hydration Therapy is nothing but consuming more than 3lirs of water after 24wks by every antenatal mother.*

Also, a down trend was observed in thromboembolic episodes. This drastic reduction of MMR in the district was due to the combined effect of SR Cannula and OHT **(Table 2)**.

SR Cannula and OHT in Andhra Pradesh: Supported by Government of Andhra Pradesh, similar hands-on training workshops were conducted at all district Head quarter hospitals of all districts of Andhra Pradesh except Vizianagaram. MMR dropped to 30 in the year 2024-25, which is the lowest in the country.

SR Cannula and OHT in Tamil Nadu: Supported by Government of Tamil Nadu and NHM, introduced SR cannula to prevent and treat PPH in all Government Health facilities in Tamil Nadu. In the month of May 2022, we conducted hands on training workshops to train the trainers from 63 Government Medical colleges at 3 centers in the state. MMR is rapidly dropped down to 35 in 2024-25.

Hands on training workshop at Bodh Gaya district (2022) of Bihar to bring down MMR: Supported by UNICEF, NHM, CARE India, we conducted hands-on training workshop from 1st to 4th August-2022 at Bodh Gaya, for doctors of all PHCs, CHCs, Referral Hospitals & Medical Colleges on

TABLE 1: Three month's performance of SR PPH suction cannula, and oral hydration therapy to prevent severe preeclampsia.

Positive result after using SR cannula (best practices) at APVVP hospitals in Chittoor district between Aug and Nov 2018									
Sl. No.	*Name of the Hospital*	*No of SRC sets available*	*Total no of deliv. occurred*	*No of N. D SRC used*	*No of C.S SRC was used*	*Total no of SRC applications*	*General comments on controlling PPH*	*Mate-renal deaths*	*Total blood units given*
1.	DHH Chittoor	6 sets	1,693	279	104	383	Control is good, but time taking	0	9
2.	AH Kuppam	3 sets	751	343	64	407	Control is good but time taking	0	6
3.	CHC Punganur	2 sets	195	3	9	12	Useful in arresting PPH	0	0
4.	AH Madanapalle	10 set	1,115	127	182	309	Useful in arresting PPH	0	7
5.	AH Srikalahast	3 sets	525	8	7	15	Saved 2 PPH cases	0	6
6.	CHC Vayalpadu	2 sets	100	43	4	47	Very useful in arresting PPH	0	0
7.	CHC Satyavedu	2 sets	59	21	1	22	Minimal blood loss	0	0
8.	CHC Piler	2 sets	690	6	7	13	Prophylactic application. Very effective in controlling PPH	0	0
9.	CHC Puttur	3 sets	162	70	12	82	Very useful in arresting PPH	0	0
10.	AH Chandragiri	2 sets	91	7	0	7	PPH Control is good	0	0
11.	CHC CG Gallu	1 set	34	5	0	5	Control is good, but time taking	0	0
12.	AH Palamaner	1 set	437	40	9	49	Minimal blood loss	0	0
13.	CHC Sodam	1 set	19	4	0	4	Applied prophylactically, minimal blood loss	0	0

Contd…

Contd...

Positive result after using SR cannula (best practices) at APVVP hospitals in Chittoor district between Aug and Nov 2018

Sl. No.	*Name of the Hospital*	*No of SRC sets available*	*Total no of deliv. occurred*	*No of N. D SRC used*	*No of C.S SRC was used*	*Total no of SRC applications*	*General comments on controlling PPH*	*Mate-renal deaths*	*Total blood units given*
14.	CHC Kalikiri	2 sets	43	35	1	36	Very good in arresting PPH. Risk reduced for M. death	0	0
15.	AH Nagari	4 sets	343	24	20	44	Applied prophylactically in Rh-ve multi. V minimal bleeding	0	0
16.	CHC V Kota	1 set	269	44	0	44	Very useful in arresting PPH	0	0
17.	CHC Thamballa Palli	1 set	56	13	9	22	Very useful in arresting PPH	0	0
18.	CHC Kothkota	2 sets	44		0	0	Useful in arresting PPH	0	0
19.	CHC Bangaru Palya	2 sets	57	2	0		Very useful	0	0
	Total	*45 sets*	*8,396*	*1,074*	*429*	*1,503*		*0*	*28*

Curtesy: Data is from DMO Chittoor.

TABLE 2: Five years' performance of SR PPH Suction Cannula, and Oral Hydration Therapy to prevent severe pre-eclampsia are shown. Very significant reduction in MMR is observed.

S. No	Year	No. of live births	No. of maternal deaths	Hemorrhagic deaths	PIH deaths	Cardiac causes for M. deaths	COVID +ve deaths	Thromboembolic episodes	MMR
Ear wise status of maternal deaths of Chittoor district									
1.	2014–15	67,833	60						88
2.	2015–16	63,696	60						94
3.	2016–17	58,221	46						79
4.	2017–18	58,683	47	9	16	1	0	2	83
SR PPH Suction cannula and OHT started in August 2018									
5.	2018–19	60,101	30	7	10	2	0	3	50
6.	2019–20	61,464	20	2	10	1	0	1	32.5
7.	2020–21	63,637	27	7	4	1	2	2	42
8.	2021–22	66,892	31	3	3	3	10	1	46
9.	2022–23	29,249	9	0	1	1	0	1	33.3

Curtesy: Data is from DMO Chittoor.

SR cannula application to prevent and treat PPH. MANUAL SUCTION PUMPS were distributed to all participating PHCs.

Hands on Training Workshop at Bidar, Karnataka State (2024)

Training was conducted for doctors of all PHCs, CHCs, Referral Hospitals & Medical Colleges of Bidar district. Supported by Government of Karnataka.

Now, Entire Kerala, Tamil Nadu, Andhra Pradesh and major hospitals in Karnataka are using this cannula to prevent and treat PPH. Kerala Federation (KFOG) included SR cannula in to its Obstetric protocols to prevent and treat PPH. We can observe, a very significant reduction in MMR to around 30 in all south Indian states. The MMR of AP has come down to 30 that is the lowest in the country, which was never before.

KEY TAKE-HOME MESSAGES

- Safe, life-saving, and fertility saving device, very useful in low resource settings.
- High success rates often outperforming intrauterine balloon tamponade. Easy to learn the technique. even staff nurses can be trained.
- Suction cannula system can be organized just within 2 minutes time, and the bleeding can be stopped just within 2–3 minutes
- Powerful global negative pressure inside the uterine cavity, assists the natural physiological mechanisms of contraction and retraction to stop atonic bleeding.
- This is a physical method, do not depend on biological factors for its action. Do not fail when applied properly.
- Works well even with complete atony of uterus. No need for tamponade test
- Cannula system works well even in cases of coagulation failure.
- For best results, Cannula should be used as a first defense, not as a last resort after losing Liters of blood.
- SR Cannula, can also be used for bleeding after MTP or vesicular mole extraction
- SR Cannula, can also be used for transporting the women to higher medical centers
- When cannula inserted, we should see all the holes of cannula should stay inside cervix.
- Cannula should not be used in association with any other devices like balloons and clamps.
- Highly cost effective, autoclavable and reusable device.

SUGGESTED READING

1. Damor P, Maheshwari S, Singh S. Role of SR vacuum cannula as novel technique for atonic PPH management study at Pannadhay Rajkiya Mahila Chikitsalaya and RNT Medical College, Udaipur. Int J Reprod Contracept Obstet Gynecol. 2021;0:4150-6.
2. Hemmanur SR, Samyuktha Illa S. Prophylactic SRPPH suction cannula application for high-risk women for atonic PPH. IOSR J Dental and Medical Sci. 2019;18(4):23-7.

3. Kamat AV, Suresh S. A Clinical Trial of Oral Hydration Therapy for the Management of Very Preterm Non-severe Preeclampsia. J South Asian Feder Obstetr Gynaecol. 2023;15(6):679-82.
4. Meshram PS, Kubde AR, Kothalkar VS, Veerendrakumar CM. Role of slow decompression, injection Carbetocin and Samarth Ram cannula for preventing postpartum haemorrhage in a patient of acute severe polyhydramnios. Int J Res Med Sci 2023;11:1827-9.
5. Mohanapriya S, Priyanka K. Prospective study to analyse effectiveness of Samartharam suction canula as a preventive strategy for postpartum haemorrhage in high-risk mothers at a teaching hospital over a period of one year. Int J Reprod Contracept Obstet Gynecol. 2025;14:467-72.
6. Paily VP, Ambujam K, Thomas B. (2012). Why Mothers Die, Kerala 2006–09. Second Report of Confidential Review of Maternal Deaths. [online] Available from https://www.kfogkerala.com/media_files/kfog-3j7780.pdf [Last accessed December, 2025].
7. Purwosunu Y, Sarkoen W, Arulkumaran S, Segnitz J. Control of postpartum hemorrhage using vacuum-induced uterine tamponade. Obstet Gynecol. 2016;128(1):33-6.
8. Raghuwanshi N, Sirsam S, Tambe S. A comparison of the effectiveness of Samarthram vacuum suction cannula with uterotonic drugs as primary management in cases of atonic PPH at tertiary care centre: a randomized clinical trial. Int J Reprod Contracept Obstet Gynecol. 2025;14:3327.
9. Ram HS, Dommety S. A case of Couvelaire uterus with coagulation dysfunction saved successfully with SR PPH suction cannula. Trop J Obstet Gynaecol. 2020;37:195-7.
10. Samartharam H, Ram SHS, Ram S, Panicker V. Vacuum retraction of uterus for the management of atonic postpartum haemorrhage. IOSR J Dent Med Sci. 2014;13(11):15-19.
11. Samartharam RH, SamyuktaS I, Nagasree V. Oral hydration therapy for the management of very preterm preeclampsia. IOSR J Dental Med Sci. 2016;15(11):3-41.
12. Sharma JC, Kollabathula P, Jindal S, Anupma A, Sarkar A, Jaggarwal S, et al. Application of a negative intrauterine pressure suction device for prophylactic management of atonic postpartum haemorrhage: A quality improvement study. Cureus. 2023;15(7):42631.
13. Suarez S, Conde-Agudelo A, Borovac-Pinheiro A, Suarez-Rebling D, Eckardt M, Theron G, et al. Uterine balloon tamponade for treatment of postpartum hemorrhage: systematic review and meta-analysis. Am J Obstet Gynecol. 2020;222(4):293.e1-293.e52
14. WHO. (2025). Trends in Maternal Mortality 2000-2023: Estimates by WHO, UNICEF, UNFPA, World Bank Group and UNDESA/Population Division. [online] Available from https://www.who.int/publications/i/item/9789240108462 [Last accessed December, 2025].

6 CHAPTER

Newer Invention in Compression Sutures

Mahesh Gupta

INTRODUCTION

Postpartum hemorrhage (PPH) is defined as bleeding of 500 mL or more within 24 h of delivery. PPH can be considered even if women become hemodynamically unstable due to the minor blood loss. In India, PPH has been reported as a major cause of maternal mortality, accounting for approximately 38% of maternal deaths.

In 1997, Christopher B-Lynch devised an innovative technique to manage uncontrolled PPH. Since then, several modifications in this technique have been published; however, none of them have a successful outcome in all patients. B-Lynch remains the standard suturing technique for the management of uncontrolled PPH. However, several concerns have been raised regarding the B-Lynch technique. Firstly, the uterine wall is punctured with a needle six times which may further provoke bleeding. Secondly, potential risks of blood entrapment, cavity occlusion, and infections cannot be overlooked as B-Lynch suture technique involves transfixation of the uterus from front to back in order to place the suture.

Due to inadequate medical facilities in developing countries like India, suturing technique complications might lead to emergency hysterectomy or maternal mortality. Herein, a simple and effective COMOC-MG (Compression Of Myometrium and OCclusion of uterine artery by Dr. Mahesh Gupta) stitch that combines uterine artery ligation with the concept of B-Lynch technique is described, for the control of life-threatening PPH using three cases. Polyglycolic acid double strand suture with 80 mm long straight taper point needle and 50-mm half circle round bodied needle **(Fig. 1)** was used in this technique. The name COMOC-MG is a registered trademark (ID: 3,175,301) of Mahesh Gopichand Gupta and is valid till 02 February 2026.

SURGICAL TECHNIQUE

The following steps are involved in the competent application of the COMOC-MG stitch **(Figs. 2A to F)**:

1. Informed consent was obtained before the surgical procedure.

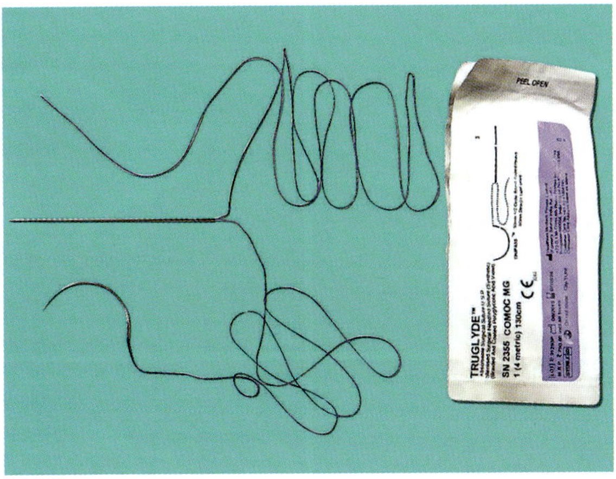

Fig. 1: The needle and thread used in this COMOC-MG stitch.

2. The patients were placed in the Lloyd Davies position for the procedure with legs apart and no head-down tilt, so that vaginal bleeding could be assessed.
3. Appropriately sized Pfannenstiel incision was used to open the abdomen.
4. After delivery, the uterus was exteriorized and inspected for bleeding sites directly while the caesarean wound was still open.
5. The procedure used for COMOC-MG stitch technique was as follows: (A) a 80 mm long straight taper point needle with polyglycolic acid double strand suture (Truglyde®, Healthium Medtech Pvt Ltd) was used to puncture the uterus 3 cm below and 3 cm medial from the lower cut edge of the uterus in the case of caesarean section or 3 cm medial from lateral edge of uterus at the isthmus, in the case of normal delivery. (B) The needle was taken out from the posterior wall after inserting it into the anterior wall at the same level. (C) The loop around the eye of the needle was cut to obtain two free limbs posteriorly and two free limbs anteriorly. Out of anterior two limbs, one has the curved needle attached to it. (D) Then, both free limbs of one strand (from double strand) were tied by a knot at the top of uterus as Heyman's suture. In Heyman's technique, two vertical sutures are placed and tied on each side of the fundus of the uterus to prevent slippage of the knot. (E) The second strand of suture material with the round body needle was now passed to the avascular area of broad ligament just below the cut edge of uterus at the same level on the posterior aspect. (F) Both the limbs of the second suture strand were also tied firmly to occlude the uterine artery. (G) The similar procedure was then repeated on the left **(Fig. 3)**.
6. The uterus was kept in an anteflexed position by an assistant, and the suture was pulled using a moderate tension to hold the uterus in

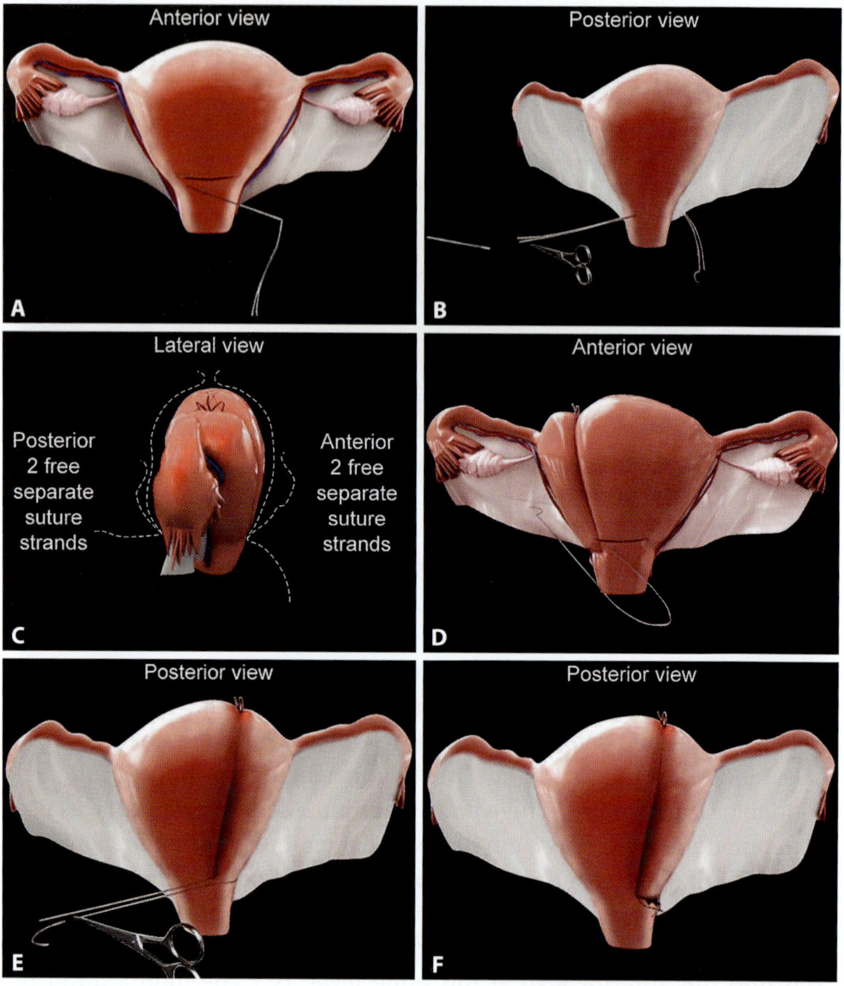

Figs. 2A to F: COMOC-MG stitch. *Notes:* (A) 80 mm long straight taper point needle is inserted into the uterus from 3 cm below and 3 cm medial to the lower cut edge of the uterus; (B) The loop around the eye of the needle is cut to obtain two free limbs posteriorly and two free limbs anteriorly; (C) From double strand, one strand will make a loop on the top of uterus as Heyman's suture; (D) The second strand with round body needle will now pass to the avascular area just below the cut edge of uterus at the same level on the posterior aspect; and (E and F) both limbs of the second suture strand tied firmly to occlude the uterine artery.

the flexion position. The suture was then tied securely. During this compression, the vagina was checked for bleeding.

7. The uterus was placed back into the abdominal cavity, and sutured, and then, the abdominal wall was closed layer by layer.
8. Care was taken not to damage the bowel and the bladder.

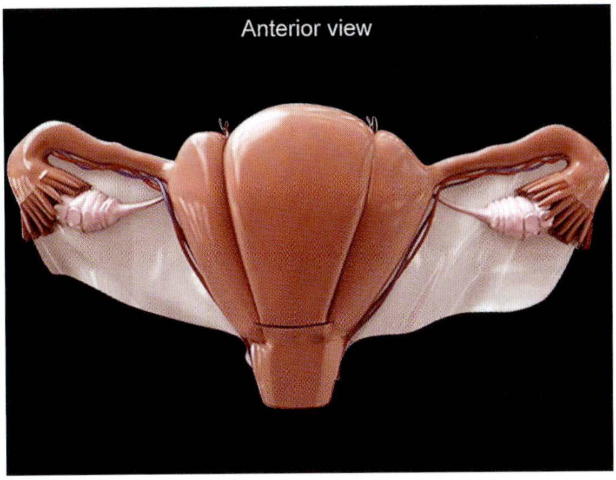

Fig. 3: COMOC-MG stitch placed on either side of the uterus.

EXPERIENCE FROM THREE CASES

COMOC-MG stitch was adopted since medical treatment such as uterine massage, bimanual compression, infusion of oxytocin (20 IU in 500 mL saline at a rate of 125 mL/h), injection of prostaglandin F2α (250 μg intramuscularly), and misoprostol (800 mg) had proved ineffective in the three cases. After suturing, there was the obvious improvement of bleeding. The duration of the procedure ranged between 4 and 5 min **(Table 1)**.

No postoperative anatomical or physiological abnormalities were seen in any of the three women. The postpartum menstrual flow and breastfeeding were normal. Ultrasound confirmed that the endometrium and ureter were normal and hysteroscopy showed a normal uterine cavity in all three women. One subsequent full-term pregnancy occurred after 6 years of this surgery in a 27-year-old woman, who delivered with repeat caesarean section.

DISCUSSION

The modified B-Lynch approach (COMOC-MG stitch described here not only successfully managed PPH during cesarean section, but also preserved fertility. This technique was used secondary to medical treatment for PPH and was successful in all the three cases. The technique is based on dual mechanism that reduced or ceased bleeding by surgical compression and ascending uterine artery branch occlusion. Adding uterine artery ligation to concept of B-Lynch technique, in COMOC-MG stitch, may help to control PPH more thoroughly during cesarean section.

COMOC-MG stitch uses a single-puncture on either side of the uterus, leaves space in the uterine cavity to allow free drainage of blood, debris, and inflammatory material, and avoids re-opening of uterine incision.

TABLE 1: Characters of patients with severe PPH treated by COMOC-MG technique.

Case no	*Age (year)*	*Gravidity and parity*	*Term (weeks of gestation)*	*Presenting diagnosis*	*Mode of delivery*	*Estimated blood loss*	*Blood transfusion (PRBC)*	*Operation time (min)*
1	36	G1P1	36 weeks	Multiple pregnancy	LSCS	300 mL (hemodynamically unstable)	–	4
2	40	G2P2	Full term	Placental previa accrete	LSCS	1,000 mL	350 mL	4
3	27	G2P2	39 weeks	Obstructed labor	LSCS	1,000 mL	700 mL	5

(LSCS: lower segment caesarian section; PRBC: packed red blood cell)

So, this technique allows conservation of the uterus and fertility. The success rate is in line with previous studies reporting successful preservation of the uterus in cases with atonic PPH. If the COMOC-MG technique fails, one can still resort to balloon therapy.

This technique can be applied for therapeutic and pro- phylactic purposes. It should be attempted as early as possible to maximize its success in women at risk of PPH. The simplicity, practicality, safety, and ease of application render this technique very efficient and reliable. Also, the learning of this modified technique requires less time as it involves the use of single puncture on either side of the uterus and can be performed in a short duration of time with limited resources. This modified suturing technique also prevents the development of undue pressure on the suture lines as no intrauterine fluid collection occurred post-operatively with this technique. Therefore, it should be considered a procedure of choice if previous medical treatment does not control atonic PPH and certainly before any radical surgery is considered.

CONCLUSION

The COMOC-MG stitch is a valuable and safe alternative to B-Lynch or other modified B-Lynch suturing techniques for successful management of atonic PPH, while preserving fertility. However, to draw a firm conclusion concerning the efficacy of this technique compared with other modifications, future studies with optimal number of cases are required.

SUGGESTED READING

1. Hayman RG, Arulkumaran S, Steer PJ. Uterine compression sutures: surgical management of postpartum hemorrhage. Obstet Gynecol. 2002;99(3):502-6.
2. Kaveh M, Tahermanesh K, Hanjani S, Abed SM. B-Lynch plus technique for uterine conservative surgery in an asymmetric atonic uterus. Int J Gynecol Obstet. 2018;142(3):370-1.
3. Moleiro ML, Braga J, Machado MJ, Guedes-Martins L. Uterine compression sutures in controlling postpartum haemorrhage: a narrative review. Acta Méd Port. 2019;35(1):51-8.
4. Montgomery AL, Ram U, Kumar R, Jha P; Million Death Study Collaborators. Maternal mortality in India: causes and healthcare service use based on a nationally representative survey. PLoS One. 2014;9(1):e83331.
5. Zahid I. (2017). Postpartum haemorrhage. [online] Available from https://www.nhp.gov.in/disease/gynae cology-and-obstetrics/postpartum-haemorrhage [Last accessed December, 2025].

7 CHAPTER

Balloon Tamponade—Chhattisgarh Balloon

Ruby Bhatia, Mahak Singaal, Komal Bansal

INTRODUCTION

Postpartum hemorrhage (PPH) remains one of the direct cause of near miss and maternal mortality worldwide. PPH is defined as the loss of more than 500 mL of blood after vaginal delivery or 1,000 mL after cesarean section or cumulative blood loss ≥1,000 mL or blood loss with signs/symptoms of hypovolemia within 24 hours after birth. The causes of PPH can be uterine atony (accounting for 80% of all), traumatic, retained placenta, coagulopathies. PPH is red alert, to be managed by multi-disciplinary approach. In atonic PPH, medical management along with resuscitative measures is the first line management while simultaneously securing airway, breathing and circulation **(Flowchart 1)**. Balloon tamponade has emerged as a significant and life-saving technique for controlling PPH when first line medical management fails to stop the bleeding. Role of AMTSL for prevention of atonic PPH cannot be underestimated. It is mandatory for prevention of atonic PPH.

Flowchart 1: Management of PPH.

Major obstetric hemorrhage:
- Blood loss greater than 1,000 mL
- Continuing major obstetric hemorrhage or clinical shock

↓

Call for help:
- Senior midwife/obstetrician and anesthetist
- Alert haematologist
- Alert blood transfusion laboratory
- Alert consultant obstetrician on call

↓

Resuscitation:
- **A**irway
- **B**reathing
- **C**irculation
- Oxygen mask (15 l)
- Fluid balance (e.g., 2 l isotonic crystalloid, 1.5 l colloid)
- Blood transfusion (O RhD-negative or group-specific blood)
- Blood products (FFP, PLT, cryoprecipitate, factor VIIa)
- Keep patient warm

This chapter explores the role of balloon tamponade in the management of PPH, including the rationale for its use, types of devices available, clinical techniques, indications, advantages, challenges, and outcomes.

PATHOPHYSIOLOGY OF POSTPARTUM HEMORRHAGE

A major contributing factor is *uterine atony* where the uterus fails to contract effectively after childbirth, leaving blood vessels uncompressed and contributing to excessive blood loss. Other factors contributing to PPH include:

- Genital tract trauma
- Retained placenta
- Coagulopathy

Balloon tamponade offers an alternative, conservative, minimally invasive approach to control atonic PPH, if first line medical management fails.

WHAT IS BALLOON TAMPONADE?

It is a involves the insertion of a balloon into the uterus, which is then inflated to exert pressure on the uterine walls. This compression helps to tamponade (stop) bleeding by applying sustained pressure upon the blood vessels at the placental site and promoting uterine contraction. Balloon tamponade is particularly effective in cases of uterine atony after vaginal delivery, cesarean section, aids to some extent in placenta previa but less effective in placenta accreta. It is highly effective modality to tide over critical phase while transferring patient from primary health center to secondary or tertiary care hospital for further management.

TYPES OF BALLOON TAMPONADE DEVICES

Various balloon tamponade devices have been developed over the years, with different designs, functions, and characteristics **(Fig. 1)**. The most commonly used devices include:

1. *Bakri balloon:* it is one of the most widely used balloon tamponade devices. It is a silicone catheter with an inflatable balloon that can hold up to 500 mL of fluid. The balloon is inserted into the uterine cavity through the cervix and inflated to apply pressure on the uterine walls. The Bakri balloon is flexible, easy to insert, and effective in controlling hemorrhage.
2. *Chhattisgarh balloon:* Stands out as a groundbreaking indigenous innovation—cost effective, sturdy, and easily deployable at PHC and CHC levels by all healthcare professionals after skilled training.
3. Sengstaken-Blakemore tube
4. Ebb balloon

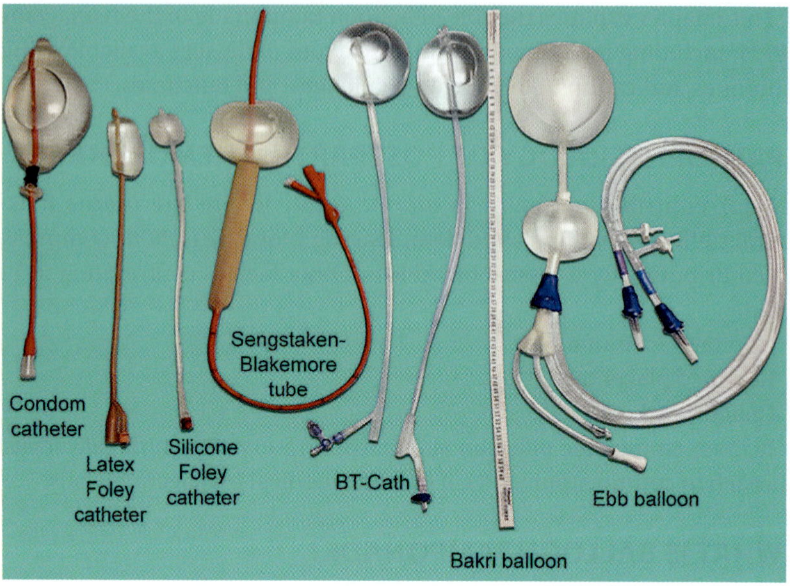

Fig. 1: Multiple types of balloon catheters have been used for intrauterine tamponade.

Chhattisgarh Balloon (Figs. 2 and 3)

Features

It uses foley's no 20/22 with connector. It requires medical-grade latex male condom. It can be inflated up to 250–500 mL. Main advantage being that it provides continuous check on bleeding from uterus as it allows for drainage as well.

Advantages

- *Highly cost effective* for government supply at PHCs/CHCs
- Simple to assemble
- Comparable efficacy to commercial balloons
- Safe referrals, minimizes surgical interventions, and reduces maternal deaths.

Insertion Technique

Balloon tamponade is inserted after first line medical management fails to control bleeding. Injectable antifibrinolytics (tranexamic acid) 1–2 g is given in management of PPH. The procedure is performed after high risk informed consent, under complete asepsis, and careful monitoring of the patient is essential. Continuous resuscitative measures, uterotonics and adequate blood and blood products are arranged.

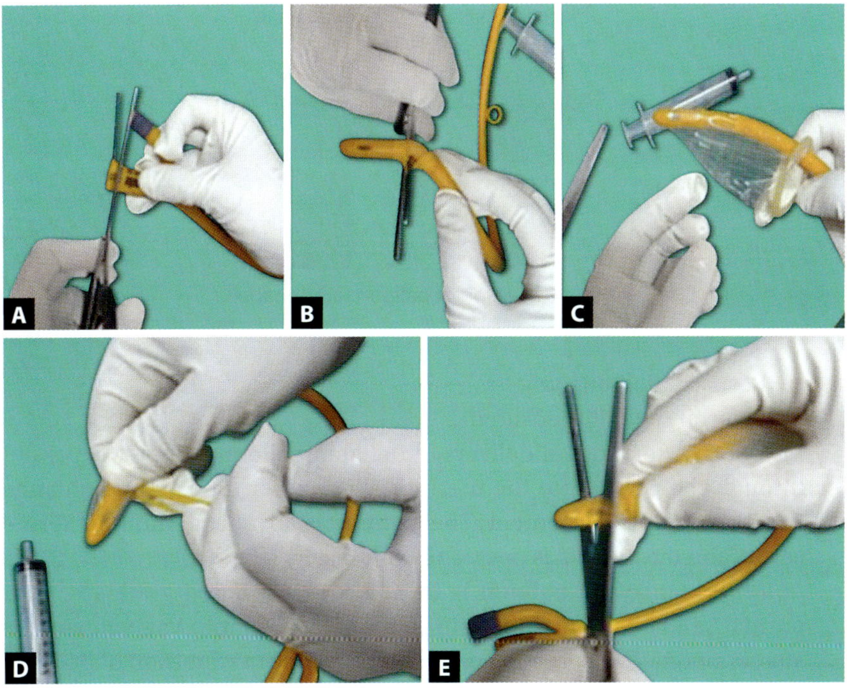

Figs. 2A to E: (A) Cutting two rings from the drainage tube of Foley's catheter; (B) Excision of the bulb of catheter after inflation with 2–5 mL of air; (C) Rolling of condom over catheter; (D) Tying condom to catheter using the rings twice around both the ends of condom leaving 1.5–2 cm of condom on either end; (E) Excision of the tip of Foley's along with the blind end of condom together 0.5 cm away from the tied ring. Leaving both the rings with CG Balloon.

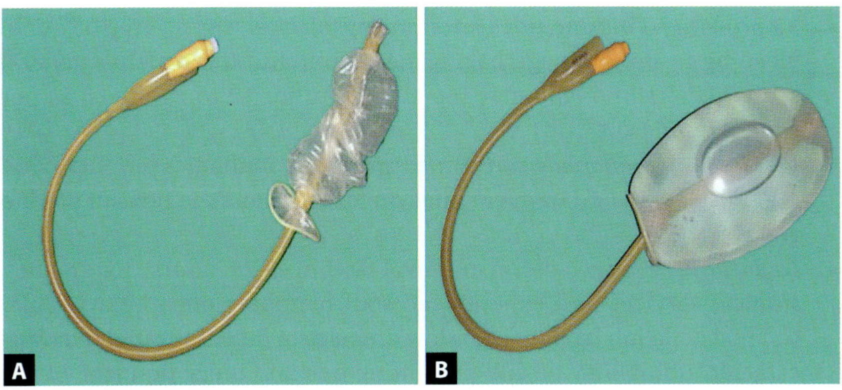

Figs. 3A and B: CG Balloon—(A) before inflation and (B) after inflation.

- *Preparation and pre-requisites:*
  - Lithotomy position, cervix examined
  - Trauma excluded, placenta expelled

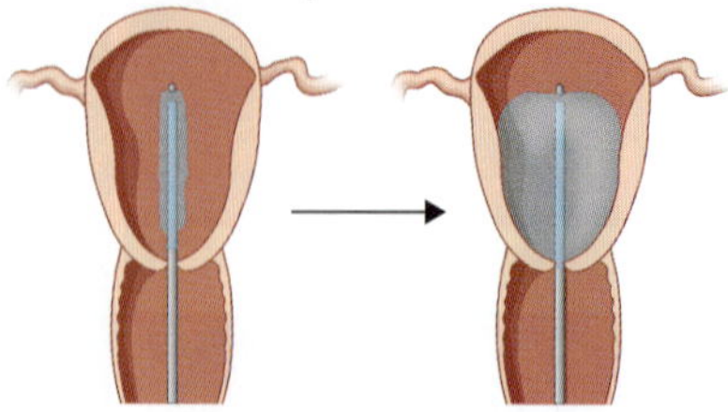

Fig. 4: Insertion of balloon tamponade.

  - Resuscitation ongoing
  - Referral capability ensured
- *Insertion:* After vaginal delivery, a deflated balloon catheter is passed through the cervix into the uterine cavity under ultrasound guidance to ensure proper placement. The catheter is advanced into the uterine cavity, and the balloon is positioned mid-cavity **(Fig. 4)**.
- *Inflation:* Once the balloon is in place, it is inflated gradually with normal saline (room temperature) up to 250–500 mL. Vaginal packing after tamponade insertion is mandatory to prevent expulsion of balloon. Attach a collection bag, ideally with a flowmeter to the drainage port. Mark the level of fundus to facilitate post tamponade monitoring.
- *Tamponade test:* Positive if bleeding stops when the balloon is partially or completely filled. Negative if bleeding fails to stop with maximum balloon filling. Cessation of bleeding from the lower segment often occurs between 250 and 300 mL of instillation, but more fluid (>500 mL) may be required to effectively stop bleeding in cases of uterine atony.
- *Monitoring:* This includes monitoring of vital signs, uterine tone, bleeding in the drainage bag, urine output and the patient's general status. The tamponade may remain in situ for 12 to 24 hours, as per clinical response.
- *Postballoon tamponade care:* Broad spectrum antibiotics prophylactics. Administer standard oxytocin infusion for 6–12 hours to prevent uterine atony.
- *Deflation:* Ensure balloon removal within 4–24 hours. Emergency surgical services and experienced staff members must be available. Gradual deflation balloon with slow drainage of fluid. For rapid removal-catheter tubing may be cut, permitting free and quick drainage of the fluid.

Indications for Balloon Tamponade

1. Atonic PPH with failure of first line medical management
2. PPH with low lying placenta/placenta previa.

3. Conservative management
4. Temporary measure before surgery
5. Temporary measure while patient transfer from primary to secondary/tertiary care hospital.

Benefits of Balloon Tamponade

1. *Simple and low cost:* Compared to surgical interventions, balloon tamponade is simple to perform, cost effective and can be done in most healthcare settings.
2. *Minimally invasive:* Balloon tamponade is non-invasive procedure. It allows for control of bleeding while avoiding surgical intervention in 80% of cases.
3. Preservation of fertility
4. *Effectiveness:* Balloon tamponade has been shown to be effective in managing uterine atony, with success rates of 80-90% after vaginal delivery, c-section and placenta previa.

COMPLICATIONS AND CHALLENGES

1. *Discomfort:* Balloon tamponade can cause discomfort or pain, particularly if the balloon is inflated too quickly or to too high a volume.
2. *Infection:* It is essential to use strict aseptic technique during insertion and to monitor the patient for signs of infection, including fever and uterine tenderness.
3. *Uterine perforation/rupture:* Due to improper technique of insertion of balloon tamponade/over-inflation, although this is a rare complication (<2%). Monitoring for signs of uterine rupture, such as severe abdominal pain or hemodynamic instability, is critical.
4. *Failure to control bleeding:* Balloon tamponade may not be effective in 10–15% atonic PPH cases or if coagulopathy has already set in or if genital trauma has not been ruled out.

OUTCOMES AND EFFECTIVENESS

The effectiveness of balloon tamponade in controlling PPH is well-documented, with success rates of 80–90% in cases of uterine atony. The technique has been associated with lower rates of surgical intervention, uterine artery embolization and peripartum hysterectomy, maternal near miss and mortality.

Outcomes may vary depending on the severity of the hemorrhage, the underlying cause, and timely intervention. Early recognition and prompt use of balloon tamponade, along with appropriate monitoring and follow-up care, contribute to better outcomes.

CARRY HOME MESSAGES

- AMTSL is mandatory for prevention of atonic PPH.
- Balloon tamponade is the mainstay measure to control atonic PPH in 80–90% cases.
- Its cost-effectiveness, minimally invasive nature, ability to preserve fertility, and effectiveness in controlling bleeding makes it an important option for clinicians managing PPH.
- It is lifesaving modality in management of atonic PPH, if first line medical management fails.
- High risk informed consent is mandatory while simultaneously managing a patient with PPH.
- Adequate blood and blood products must be ready in the blood bank.
- Balloon tamponade should be inserted before coagulopathy sets in and after traumatic PPH has been ruled out.
- Simultaneous resuscitative measures, prophylactic antibiotics and uterotonics are integral part of balloon tamponade insertion.

SUGGESTED READING

1. Anderson JM, Etches D. Non-pneumatic anti-shock garment and uterine balloon tamponade: a review. Best Pract Res Clin Obstet Gynaecol. 2008;22(6): 1047-61.
2. Bakri Y, Amri A, Abdul Jabbar F. Tamponade-balloon for obstetrical bleeding. Int J Gynaecol Obstet. 2001;74(2):139-42.
3. Burke TF, Danso-Bamfo S, Akoko L. The ESM-UBT package for postpartum hemorrhage control in resource-limited settings. BJOG. 2016;123(9):1532-9.
4. Escobar MF, Nassar AH, Theron G, Barnea ER, Nicholson W, Ramasauskaite D, et al.; FIGO Safe Motherhood and Newborn Health Committee. FIGO recommendations on the management of postpartum haemorrhage 2022. Int J Gynaecol Obstet. 2022;157(Suppl 1):3-50.
5. FIGO Safe Motherhood and Newborn Health Committee. Uterine balloon tamponade for the management of postpartum hemorrhage within health systems. Int J Gynaecol Obstet. 2021;152(3):408-11.
6. Gupta S, Manyonda IT. Uterine balloon tamponade for postpartum haemorrhage: a review. Women's Health (Lond).2014;10(6):573-82.
7. Pendleton A, Natarajan A, Awoonor-Williams J. Uterine balloon tamponade for uncontrolled postpartum hemorrhage in low-resource settings: a systematic review. Int J Gynaecol Obstet. 2016;134(2):124-9.
8. Suarez S, Conde-Agudelo A, Borovac-Pinheiro A, Suarez-Rebling D, Eckardt M, Theron G, et al. Uterine balloon tamponade for postpartum hemorrhage: a systematic review and meta-analysis. Am J Obstet Gynecol. 2020;222(4):293.e1-293.e52.
9. Tindell K, Garfinkel R, Abu-Haydar E, Ahn R, Burke TF, Conn K, et al. Uterine balloon tamponade for the treatment of postpartum hemorrhage: a systematic review. Obstet Gynecol. 2013;120(1):5-14.
10. World Health Organization. WHO recommendations for the prevention and treatment of postpartum haemorrhage. Geneva: WHO; 2017.

8 CHAPTER

Paily's Clamps to Control Obstetric Hemorrhage

VP Paily

INTRODUCTION

There are several methods to arrest obstetric hemorrhage. The most basic step was and still is, to apply pressure directly at the bleeding site. Typically we use direct pressure as in bimanual compression on uterus or aortic compression. But, for how long can we do it consistently and is it effective in situations like placenta accreta spectrum. Those with more facilities developed Interventional Radiology assisted procedure like intra-arterial balloon. If vascular surgeons are available, they would dissect the vessel and cross clamp it with atraumatic clamps. But how practical and available are these steps is anybody's guess. It is after considering all these factors that we developed the following clamps to tackle obstetric hemorrhage. The basic tenets we followed in developing these clamps were that they should be affordable and usable by the practicing obstetricians. A brief note about the recently developed clamps is given below.

THE AORTA CLAMP

This clamp was developed when we started to face more and more cases of placenta accreta spectrum (PAS). The existing recommendation at that time was to use intra-aortic balloon catheter to control the bleeding during surgery for PAS. For most of the centers in Kerala, this was not a feasible option. We conceived the idea of an atraumatic clamp which can be applied by the operating obstetrician without the aid of a vascular surgeon. The clamp was tried in cadaver dissection models and then in real cases of PAS after getting ethical clearance and informed consent from the patients **(Fig. 1)**. This clamp is patented in India, in my name and its use in PAS cases was published in the FIGO journal. This clamp is used during surgery for PAS, in almost all the major centers in Kerala **(Fig. 2)**.

TRANSVAGINAL UTERINE ARTERY CLAMP

We are faced with more and more cases of lower segment PPH after the advent of cervical ripening using mechanical methods like Foley catheter and prostaglandins. The existing methods like suction canula to control the bleeding from the uterus do not work in the case of lower segment PPH.

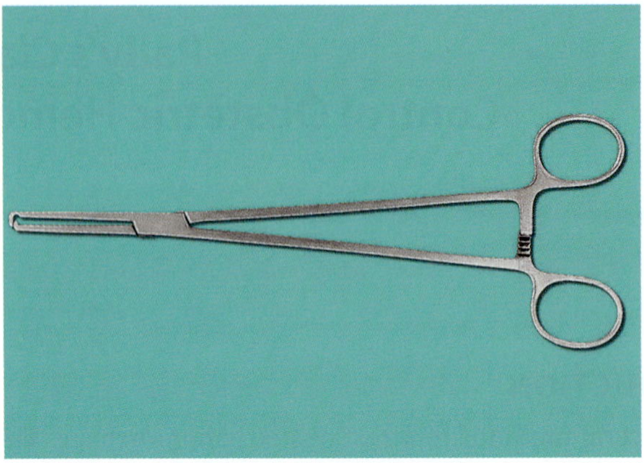

Fig. 1: The aorta clamp.

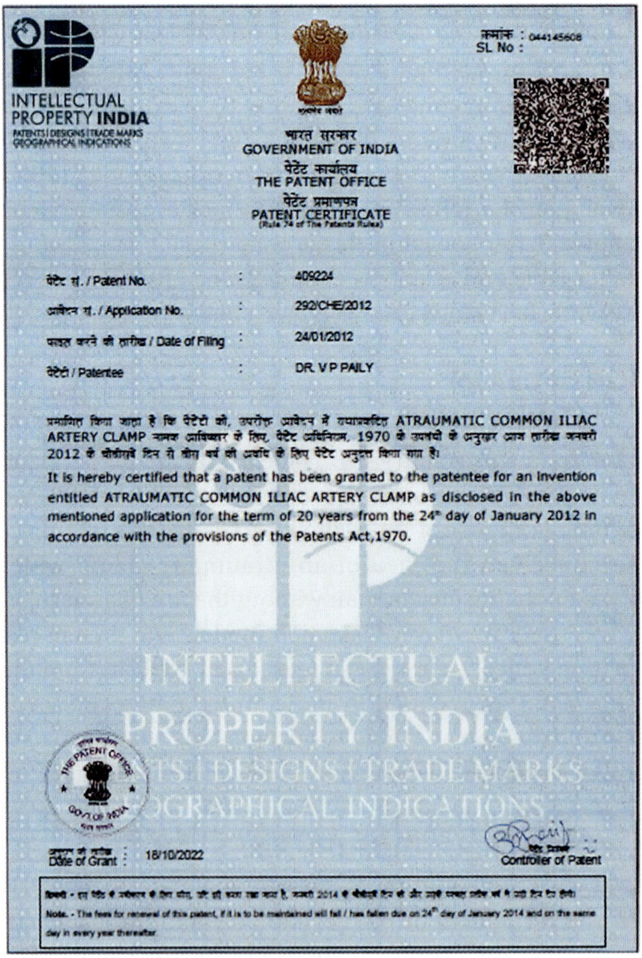

INTELLECTUAL PROPERTY INDIA
PATENTS | DESIGNS | TRADE MARKS
GEOGRAPHICAL INDICATIONS

क्रमांक : 044145608
SL No :

भारत सरकार
GOVERNMENT OF INDIA
पेटेंट कार्यालय
THE PATENT OFFICE
पेटेंट प्रमाणपत्र
PATENT CERTIFICATE
(Rule 74 of The Patents Rules)

पेटेंट सं. / Patent No.	:	409224
आवेदन सं. / Application No.	:	292/CHE/2012
फाइल करने की तारीख / Date of Filing	:	24/01/2012
पेटेंटी / Patentee	:	DR. V P PAILY

प्रमाणित किया जाता है कि पेटेंटी को, उपरोक्त आवेदन में यथाप्रकटित ATRAUMATIC COMMON ILIAC ARTERY CLAMP नामक आविष्कार के लिए, पेटेंट अधिनियम, 1970 के उपबंधों के अनुसार आज तारीख जनवरी 2012 के चौबीसवें दिन से बीस वर्ष की अवधि के लिए पेटेंट अनुदत्त किया गया है।

It is hereby certified that a patent has been granted to the patentee for an invention entitled ATRAUMATIC COMMON ILIAC ARTERY CLAMP as disclosed in the above mentioned application for the term of 20 years from the 24th day of January 2012 in accordance with the provisions of the Patents Act,1970.

अनुदान की तारीख
Date of Grant : 18/10/2022

Controller of Patent

टिप्पणी - [illegible]

Note. - The fees for renewal of this patent, if it is to be maintained will fall / has fallen due on 24th day of January 2014 and on the same day in every year thereafter.

Fig. 2: Intellectual property India certificate.

Hence, I developed an atraumatic clamp that can be applied vaginally to occlude the uterine arteries, in cases of PPH, especially in the low resource settings. The transvaginal uterine artery clamp (TVUAC) with the 'L' shape was introduced and its use is published in the European Journal **(Fig. 3)**.

THE 'T' CLAMP

As a modification of the TVUAC, which was 'L' shaped, we developed the 'T' clamp which was smaller in the terminal part and easier to apply transvaginally. This clamp is recommended in place of the 'L' clamp and we train even the labor room nurses to apply it **(Fig. 4)**.

TRANSABDOMINAL 'T' CLAMP

Often there is the need to immediately arrest bleeding from the angles or the edges of the uterine wounds, even before the placenta is delivered.

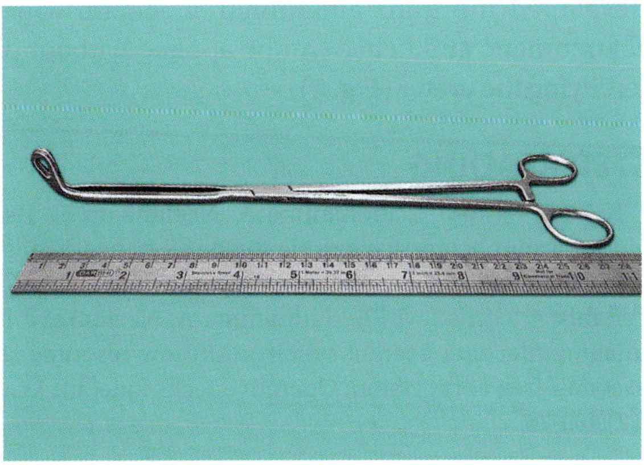

Fig. 3: Transvaginal uterine artery clamp (TVUAC).

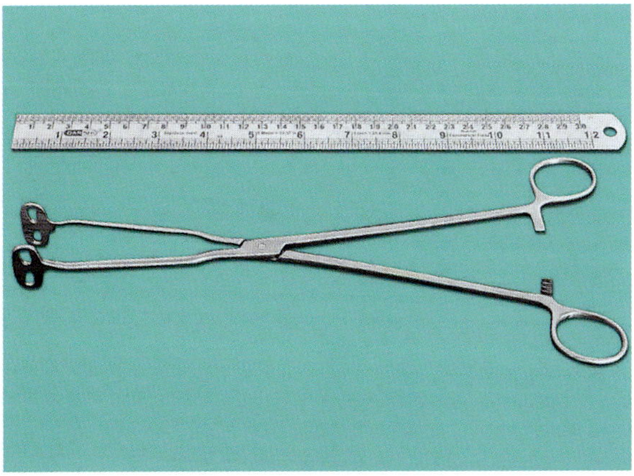

Fig. 4: The 'T' clamp.

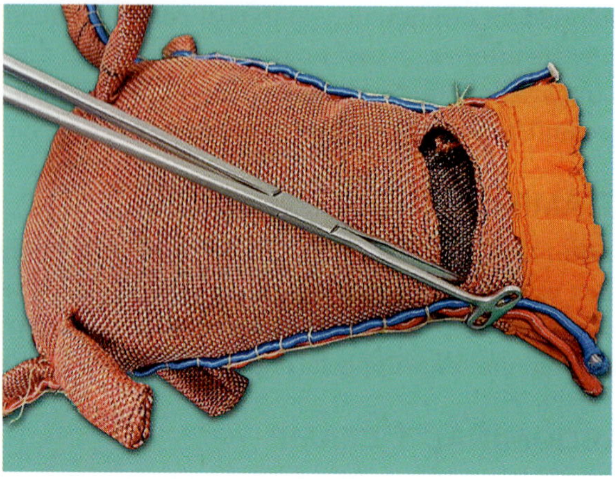

Fig. 5: Transabdominal 'T' clamp.

Hence, we developed the trans abdominal 'T' clamp which is shorter in length and atraumatic and hence can be applied without dissecting the bladder or identifying the ureter **(Fig. 5)**.

SUGGESTED READING

1. Paily VP, Raj GR, Sidhik A, Sudhamma A, Neelankavil JJ, Usha MG, et al. Arresting postpartum hemorrhage using the novel trans-vaginal uterine artery clamp. Eur J Obstet Gynecol Reprod Biol. 2022;272:6-15.
2. Paily VP, Sidhik A, Girijadevi RR, Sudhamma A, Neelankavil JJ, Menon UG, et al. Managing placenta accreta spectrum in low resource setting using a novel dissection-free aorta clamp: Operative technique. Int J Gynecol Obstet. 2022;158(2):469-75.

9 CHAPTER

Coagulopathy and Postpartum Hemorrhage

Charmila Ayyavoo

INTRODUCTION

The National Health Mission, India has stated in 2024 that postpartum hemorrhage (PPH) is the cause for 38% of maternal deaths. PPH can be due to the 4 Ts like tone, trauma, tissue and thrombin.

ETIOLOGY

Coagulopathy in PPH may be due to dilutional causes, general consumption of clotting factors, local consumption of coagulation factors, or due to excessive fibrinolysis. Dilutional coagulopathy occurs when there is replacement of blood loss with crystalloids and colloids, instead of blood and there is dilution of coagulation factors and platelets. General consumption occurs in amniotic fluid embolism (AFE), infection, severe abruption, and preeclampsia. Local consumption of coagulation factors occurs in abruption of the placenta, atonic uterus, retained and adherent placenta. Early coagulopathy is more common in AFE and placental abruption. It is not common in uterine atony and trauma to the genital tract. The commonest causes of coagulopathy in PPH are late identification of massive blood loss and underestimation of blood loss.

PATHOLOGY OF COAGULOPATHY

Tone

There are three mechanisms by which coagulopathy occurs in an atonic uterus. They are mechanical, cellular, and secondary changes of coagulation. When there is atonicity, the uterus does not contract adequately and the spiral arteries and sinusoids remain dilated and open. Blood from the bed of the placenta flows briskly into the uterine cavity. The "physiologic ligature" is lost and there is ongoing hemorrhage. The cellular changes are fatigue of the uterine muscle which may occur due to prolonged labor, over distension of the uterus due to multiple pregnancy, polyhydramnios, and macrosomia, or infection which can cause reduction in intracellular calcium and ATP, and actin-myosin crossbridge cycling. There may be desensitization of the oxytocin receptors which can reduce uterine muscle contractility.

This happens when there is prolonged exposure to high dose oxytocin. Mediators of inflammation in infection, and preeclampsia can disrupt calcium signaling and prostaglandin synthesis needed for uterine contraction. The third mechanism in atonic uterus is because of the changes in coagulation. Prolonged bleeding can cause depletion of coagulation factors and platelets which will aggravate the bleeding.

Trauma

Excess bleeding depletes coagulation factors and platelets leading to coagulopathy. Replacement with fluids instead of blood also depletes coagulation factors.

Tissue

Retained placenta can cause atonicity and there can be local consumption of coagulation factors resulting in coagulopathy.

Thrombin

Injury to the placenta releases tissue thromboplastins into the maternal circulation. There is also endothelial damage which can cause general activation of the coagulation cascade. There is rapid reduction in coagulation factors and platelets, deposition of fibrin in microcirculation and thrombosis of placenta resulting in depletion of fibrin, thrombocytopenia, and coagulation failure. This process is very severe in concealed abruption with intrauterine fetal death.

Disseminated Intravascular Coagulation

Obstetric cause for disseminated intravascular coagulation (DIC) is very rare. It can occur in severe hypertensive disorder in pregnancy, retained stillbirth, sepsis, amniotic fluid embolism, severe abruption, acute fatty liver of pregnancy, and unrecognized severe PPH. The condition is diagnosed by reducing platelet levels, and fibrinogen with a rise in fibrin degradation products (FDPs). In pregnancy, FDPs are increased at term and there is no definite cut off value for diagnosis of DIC during PPH. It is very difficult to differentiate in acute bleeding between DIC and the other causes of coagulopathy. There is end organ micro-vascular thrombosis in DIC and prompt treatment is crucial to prevent morbidity.

MONITORING OF HEMOSTATIC INSTABILITY

1. Clinical observation
2. Laboratory-based prothrombin time (PT), activated partial thromboplastin time (aPPT), Clauss fibrinogen, platelet count
3. Point of care testing (POCT)

Single measurements are not enough in the management of obstetric induced coagulopathy. Repeated measurements at appropriate intervals are needed to understand the trending of the disorder.

New Point-of-Care Tests

Point-of-care tests (POCT) are more advantageous than traditional tests. Thromboelastography (TEG) and thromboelastometry (ROTEM®) are viscoelastic tests which can be done on whole or citrated blood. They can measure clot kinetics and strength from formation to fibrinolysis. POCT is available for platelet testing now.

INTERPRETATION OF INVESTIGATIONS AND MANAGEMENT IN COAGULOPATHY

Fibrinogen falls earlier than other coagulation factors during PPH and may be low even if there is normal PT/aPTT. Fibrinogen >4 g/L is associated with a low rate of progression to severe PPH. (ideal is >2). Fibrinogen can be replaced using cryoprecipitate or fibrinogen concentrate. The dose should be calculated based on the measured and target fibrinogen. Two pools (10 packs) of cryoprecipitate can increase fibrinogen by about 1 g/L. Fibrinogen concentrate at a dose of 60 mg/kg can increase fibrinogen by 1 g/L. If fibrinogen correction is done earlier, the need for blood transfusions is decreased rapidly. In severe abruption and AFE, empirical infusion with 2 pools of cryoprecipitate can be considered.

Fresh frozen plasma (FFP) can be given based on the PT/aPTT levels. If they are prolonged, FFP is given in the dose of 15 mL/kg body weight. If hemostatic tests are not available and bleeding is continuing after 4 units of RBC, four of FFP should be infused and 1:1 RBC:FFP transfusions is maintained.

Platelets should be given at levels of 75,000 to maintain a level >50,000 during ongoing PPH. Early fall in platelet levels are not commonly seen in PPH due to atonicity or trauma. The fall should be anticipated in severe HDP, gestational or other causes of thrombocytopenia, abruption, AFE, blood loss of more than 4,000 mL. There is no need to transfuse fixed ratio of platelets with packed cells and FFP. If blood tests are not available and already 8 units of packed cells and 8 units of FFP has been transfused, then two pools of cryoprecipitate and one pool of platelets are transfused.

HEMOSTATIC AGENTS IN PPH

Tranexamic acid, factor 7, fibrinogen concentrate, Desmopressin (DDAVP) and Recombinant Human Soluble Thrombomodulin (rhTM) can be tried in PPH in special circumstances.

One gram of tranexamic acid is given intravenously within 3 hours of birth if there is bleeding. A second dose can be repeated if bleeding starts again after half an hour. (RCOG) Factor 7 is given if there is active bleeding even after conventional treatment for PPH. It should be given only if the fibrinogen and platelet levels are within normal limits. The initial dose is 40–60 μg/kg. If two doses have not corrected the bleeding, it may not be useful to repeat the doses.

DDAVP is a synthetic anti diuretic hormone analog and it increases factor VIII concentrations and VWF release from endothelial cells, promoting platelet aggregation and adhesion. It is useful in DIC due to abnormal platelet activity. Recombinant Human Soluble Thrombomodulin (rhTM) is an anti-coagulant which can be tried in DIC due to sepsis. It can reduce excessive activation of thrombin.

CONCLUSION

In PPH, coagulopathy can be a cause and a consequence. The early identification, appropriate treatment, and effective escalation of management can save many maternal lives. There should be skills and drills in each maternity unit for meeting this common problem. When there is no plan in place for PPH in the labor ward and operation theatre, there may be a dramatic increase in complications which could have been averted by timely management. Coagulopathy in PPH should be anticipated by clinicians treating the mothers during delivery and an algorithm should be developed by every unit for management for an effective fall in our nation's maternal mortality and morbidity.

KEY MESSAGES

- Around 25% of cases of major obstetric hemorrhage are associated with coagulopathy.
- It can be due to consumption of clotting factors, dilution of remaining factors by fluid volume replacement, and endothelial activation from hypothermia and acidosis.
- Nature of coagulopathy depends on the cause of bleeding.
- Surgical trauma and atony cause dilutional PPH in early stage.
- Abruption and amniotic fluid embolism cause early fibrinogen loss and DIC.
- Hence etiology is very important in management.

SUGGESTED READING

1. Collins P, Abdul-Kadir R, Thachil J; Subcommittees on Women' s Health Issues in Thrombosis and Haemostasis and on Disseminated Intravascular Coagulation. Management of coagulopathy associated with postpartum hemorrhage: guidance from the SSC of the ISTH. J Thromb Haemost. 2016; 14(1):205-10.

2. Cunningham FG, Leveno KJ, Dashe JS, Hoffman BL, Spong CY, Casey BM. Williams Obstetrics, 26th Edition. Philadelphia: McGraw Hill; 2022.
3. Erez O, Othman M, Rabinovich A, Leron E, Gotsch F, Thachil J. DIC in Pregnancy - Pathophysiology, Clinical Characteristics, Diagnostic Scores, and Treatments. J Blood Med. 2022;13:21-44.
4. Gillissen A, van den Akker T, Caram-Deelder C, Henriquez DDC, Bloemenkamp KWM, van Roosmalen J, et al. Association between fluid management and dilutional coagulopathy in severe postpartum haemorrhage: a nationwide retrospective cohort study. BMC Pregnancy Childbirth. 2018;18(1):398.
5. Katz D, Beilin Y. Disorders of coagulation in pregnancy. Br J Anaesth. 2015: 115(Suppl 2):ii75-88.
6. Prevention and Management of Postpartum Haemorrhage: Green-top Guideline No. 52. BJOG. 2017;124(5):e106-49.

10 CHAPTER

Dangers of Overloading in Postpartum Hemorrhage

Jaya Tulaskar, Rashmi Kahar

INTRODUCTION

Postpartum hemorrhage (PPH) remains the leading cause of maternal mortality worldwide, particularly in low-resource settings. PPH is associated with substantial maternal morbidity and mortality. In the management of postpartum hemorrhage (PPH), aggressive fluid and blood product replacement is critical, but *fluid overload poses a significant danger*, potentially leading to serious complications like pulmonary edema, dilutional coagulopathy, and cardiac dysfunction. Fluid resuscitation is a cornerstone of PPH treatment to restore hemodynamic stability; however, excessive or injudicious administration of intravenous (IV) fluids and blood products can result in the following complications.

TRANSFUSION-RELATED ACUTE LUNG INJURY

Transfusion-related acute lung injury (TRALI), is a clinical syndrome in which there is acute, noncardiogenic pulmonary edema TRALI is best described as a clinical constellation of dyspnea and bilateral pulmonary edema that usually develops during, or within 6 h of, a transfusion. Hypoxemia, fever, hypotension, tachycardia and cyanosis also often occur. Although the symptoms usually commence within 1–2 h of transfusion, some patients can develop dyspnea as late as 48 h after transfusion (atypical TRALI). Clinical findings include exudative bilateral infiltrates on chest radiograph, no evidence of pulmonary vascular overload, and hypoxemia of SpO_2 less than 90% on room air with a ratio of the partial pressure of oxygen to a fractional inspired oxygen concentration of less than 300 mm Hg. Nearly 30% of patients will have low levels of BNP and transient leucopenia. Immediate management of TRALI is to stop the transfusion and notify the blood bank to screen the donor unit for antileukocyte antibodies, anti-HLA or anti-neutrophil-specific antibodies. Supportive measures must be taken to improve oxygenation. Although there is no specific treatment for TRALI, best practice is prevention. Once the transfusion is stopped, gradual recovery may take 2–4 days. The chest X-ray will improve within 2–5 days.

TRANSFUSION-ASSOCIATED CIRCULATORY OVERLOAD

This is a specific complication related to rapid or excessive blood product transfusion, where the circulatory system cannot handle the increased volume, leading to heart failure symptoms and respiratory distress (a form of pulmonary edema).

Differentiation of Transfusion-related Acute Lung Injury and Transfusion-associated Circulatory Overload (Fig. 1)

Transfusion-associated circulatory overload (TACO) is a simulated cardiogenic pulmonary edema as a result of altered cytokine profile, and TRALI-syndrome is a consequence of specific immunologic conflict between donor and recipient after hemotransfusion, these conditions should be differentiated in the inpatient setting, and specialists should use the full range of modern laboratory and instrumental methods **(Table 1)**.

Table 1 shows differentiating TRALI and TACO.

Figure 1 showing difference between TRALI versus TACO.

Dilutional Coagulopathy

Administering large volumes of crystalloid fluids or even packed red blood cells without balancing with plasma and platelets can dilute the patient's existing clotting factors, worsening the underlying bleeding and potentially leading to a vicious cycle of hemorrhage and resuscitation. It happens when rapid fluid/blood product replacement dilutes clotting factors and platelets, impairing the blood's ability to clot, especially with massive bleeding from causes like atony or trauma.

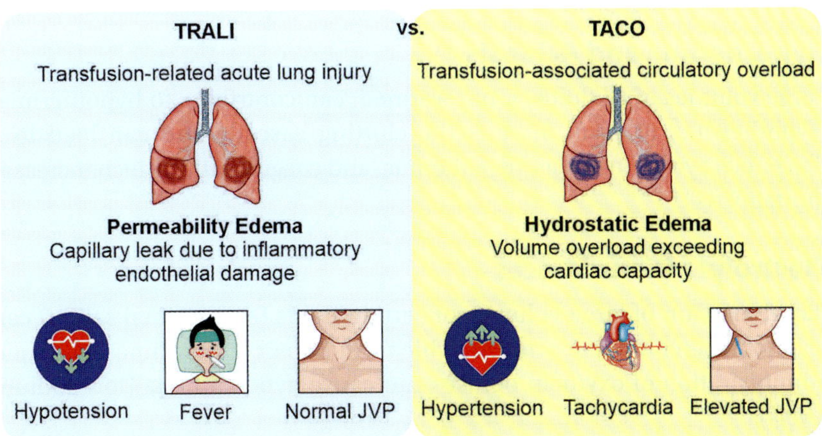

Fig. 1: TRALI versus TACO.

TABLE 1: Difference between TRALI and TACO.

Indicator	*TRALI*	*TACO*
Similar characteristics		
Chest X-ray	Diffuse bilateral infiltrates	Diffuse bilateral infiltrates
Respiratory syndrome	Dyspnea	Dyspnea
Auscultation	Wheezing	Wheezing, predominantly in the S3 segment
Different characteristics		
Body temperature	Often elevated	Often unchanged
Blood pressure	Hypotension	Hypertension
Pulmonary artery occlusion pressure	≤18 mm Hg	>18 mm Hg
Response to diuretics	Minimal	Significant
Pulmonary edema	Exudative	Transudative
White blood cell count in peripheral blood	Possible transient leucopenia	No change
Fluid balance	Normal, positive, negative	Positive

Key Features

- Decreased fibrinogen levels (hypofibrinogenemia).
- Reduced thrombin generation.
- Prolonged clotting times (PT/aPTT) and low platelets in severe cases.
- It's managed by restricting crystalloids (1–2 mL per 1 mL blood loss), using restrictive transfusion ratios (e.g., 1:1 RBC:FFP), giving tranexamic acid (TXA), and replacing fibrinogen/platelets quickly with concentrates or FFP to restore coagulation balance and stop severe bleeding.

Hypothermia and Acidosis

Large volumes of IV fluids, if not warmed, can contribute to hypothermia. Hypothermia, in turn, impairs the clotting cascade and can lead to a dangerous cycle of acidosis, hypothermia, and coagulopathy, which increases mortality risk.

Electrolyte Disturbances

Rapid infusion of large volumes of certain fluids (e.g., normal saline) can lead to hyperchloremic acidosis, which can impair kidney function. Rapid administration of oxytocin boluses can cause hyponatremia (low sodium levels).

Adverse reactions to blood transfusions, such as febrile nonhemolytic reactions, allergic reactions, acute hemolytic reactions.

Despite stringent screening measures, the risk of transfusion-transmitted infections (e.g., HIV, hepatitis B and C, bacterial infections) remains, albeit low. Infections pose a significant concern, especially in settings with inadequate blood screening protocols.

Prolonged-term transfusion can lead to iron overload in recipients. This excess iron can accumulate in organs (e.g., liver, heart, pancreas), leading to complications such as liver dysfunction, cardiac issues, endocrine disturbances, and increased oxidative stress.

Repeated exposure to transfused blood components can trigger alloimmunization, leading to the development of antibodies against certain blood antigens. This can pose challenges in finding compatible blood for future transfusions and may result in delayed hemolytic transfusion reactions.

Alterations in coagulation parameters due to prolonged-term transfusion might predispose individuals to thrombotic complications such as deep vein thrombosis (DVT) or pulmonary embolism (PE).

MANAGEMENT STRATEGIES TO AVOID OVERLOAD

Tailoring transfusion to individual patient needs while minimizing unnecessary transfusions helps prevent complications associated with excessive transfusion. Close monitoring of vital signs, hematological parameters, and clinical status before, during, and after transfusion is essential. Considering patient-specific factors, such as baseline hemoglobin levels, comorbidities, and the severity of hemorrhage, is crucial in determining the appropriate transfusion strategy.

Current best practices emphasize balanced, "damage control resuscitation" to mitigate these risks:

Massive Transfusion Protocols

When significant blood loss occurs, institutions typically initiate massive transfusion protocols (MTPs), which involve fixed ratios of packed red blood cells, fresh-frozen plasma, and platelets (commonly a 1:1:1 ratio) to prevent dilutional coagulopathy.

Flowchart 1 showing adult massive transfusion protocol.

Hypotensive Fluid Resuscitation

Permissive hypotension, also known as hypotensive fluid resuscitation, is an alternative method currently recommended as the preferred strategy for treating PPH. This more cautious approach involves restricting the use of crystalloid fluids to maintain the patient's blood pressure lower than normal to limit secondary blood loss until control of bleeding is achieved and to

Flowchart 1: Adult massive transfusion protocol.

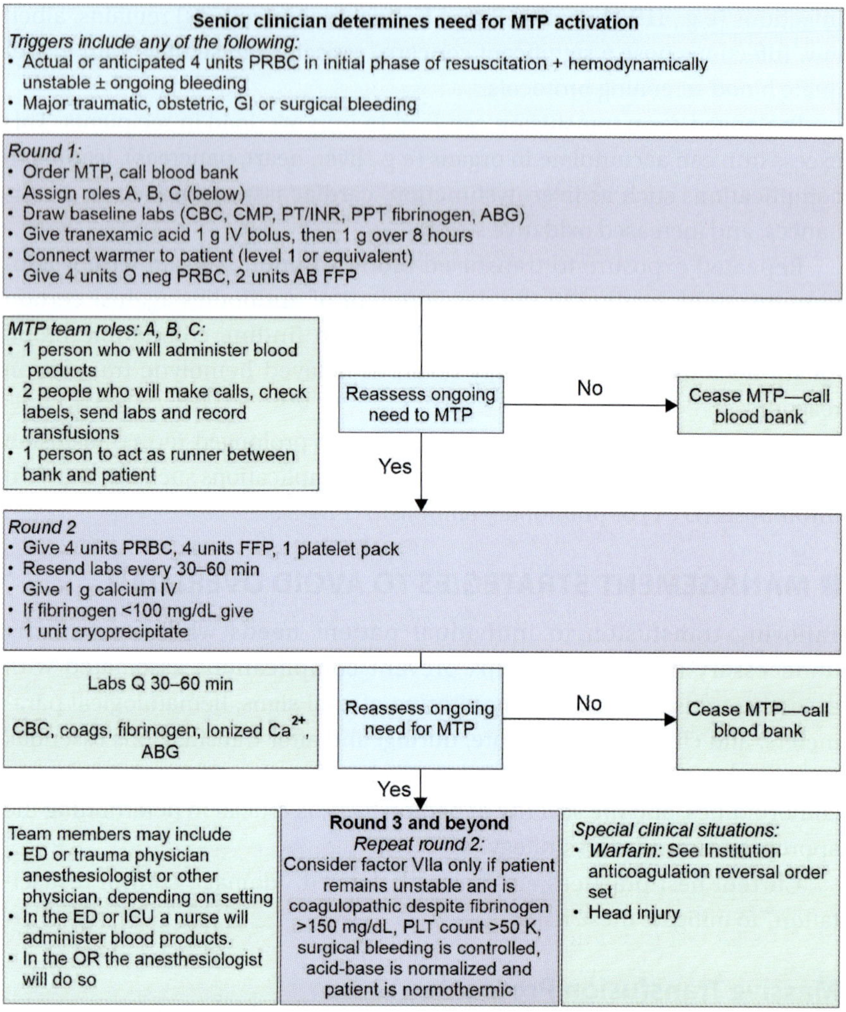

Source: Fredericks C, Kubasiak JC, Mentzer CJ, Yon JR. Massive transfusion: An update for the anesthesiologist. World J Anesthesiol. 2017;6(1):14-21.

prevent fluid overload. The aim of administering small crystalloid volumes is to provide adequate tissue perfusion and oxygen delivery to the body's tissues but reduce the risk of dilutional coagulopathy and prevent the disruption of pre-formed blood clots. Recent guidelines recommend avoiding using more than 2 liters of crystalloid solutions or 1.5 liters of colloids in the treatment of PPH before resorting to blood transfusion. In treating PPH, it is more important to rapidly replace fluids and warm the solutions than to focus on the specific type of fluid being infused.

Goals of Fluid Therapy

- Crystalloids should be followed immediately with packed red cell replacement using packed red blood cells (RBC) to restore oxygen-carrying capacity and maintain hemoglobin greater than 8 g/dL.
- To maintain systolic pressure of 80–90 mm Hg, urine output >0.5 mL/kg/h, and normal mental status. Rather than following the standard practice of fluid administration, clinicians should adjust fluid infusion to maintain a target systolic blood pressure of 80–90 mm Hg until major bleeding has been controlled. An alternative goal of fluid administration during the bleeding phase of severe postpartum hemorrhage is to achieve a low mean arterial pressure, which has been recommended to be between 50–60 mm Hg and 55–65 mm Hg.

Colloids versus Crystalloids

Colloid solutions may be used as an alternative or an adjunct to crystalloids with the assumption of its greater and longer duration of volume expansion effect. But no colloid solution has been demonstrated to be superior to crystalloids. Compared to crystalloids, colloids are more expensive and carry a greater risk of adverse effects. For the resuscitation of women with PPH, isotonic crystalloids should be used in preference to colloids. Avoid dextrans in obstetric practice as they may interfere with platelet function and cross-matching and are hazardous. Also, avoid using hydroxyethyl starch for resuscitation in major PPH.

Which Crystalloid to Give?

- Ringer's lactate and normal saline are the two most commonly used crystalloid solutions for initial fluid resuscitation. Until blood is available, infuse crystalloid at a volume that is approximately three times the estimated volume of blood loss.
- Normal saline is usually administered in a labor ward because of its easy availability, low cost, and compatibility with blood transfusions and most drugs. But the infusion of large quantities (>2 L) of normal saline can cause hyperchloremic acidosis and acute kidney injury. Ringer's lactate solution, compared to normal saline, has an electrolyte composition that more closely resembles plasma Dextrose-containing IV solutions, such as 5% dextrose or dextrose with saline, should not be used in treating PPH because the rapid infusion of these solutions can cause hyperglycemia and resultant diuresis.

BLOOD REPLACEMENT

Timely and adequate blood replacement is crucial and lifesaving in the treatment of severe PPH.

Indications of Blood Replacement

- There are no clear guidelines for determining when a red blood cell transfusion should be infused [Patients with acute hemorrhage can have normal hemoglobin, so it is important to pay close attention to the clinical evaluation.
- Common indications of red cell transfusion in PPH are:
  - Women with a hemoglobin value <6 g/dL, irrespective of symptoms.
  - Clinically severe uncontrollable postpartum hemorrhage.
  - Blood loss of 1,500 mL or more usually requires blood/pack cell transfusion.
  - Blood is usually administered to symptomatic women (maternal tachycardia >110 beats per minute, dizziness, syncope) with active bleeding, irrespective of hemoglobin status. The combination of a higher shock index (>9) and lactate levels (>4.0 mmol/L), with immediate postpartum lower hemoglobin, predicts the requirement for blood transfusion.

Selection of Blood Product

Packed red blood cells (PRBCs) are preferred for resuscitation and to avoid crystalloids-induced dilutional coagulopathy in women with massive hemorrhage. Packed red blood cells are the preferred treatment for hypovolemic shock caused by hemorrhage, and each unit can be expected to increase the hemoglobin level by about 1 gm/dL. When a large volume of transfusion is required, recommended proportionate administration of red blood cells, fresh frozen plasma (FFP), and platelets are in a 1:1:1 ratio, which resembles the replacement of whole blood.

Point-of-Care Testing

Utilizing tests like thromboelastography (TEG) and thromboelastometry demonstrated high diagnostic accuracy for hypofibrinogenemia in PPH can help clinicians more rapidly and accurately identify the need for specific blood components, optimizing replacement and avoiding unnecessary volume. The new era of thromboelastometry relies on its efficacy, practicality, reproducibility and cost-effectiveness to establish itself as the main diagnostic tool and transfusion guide in patients with severe active bleeding.

Tools Used in Point-of-Care Testing

In clinical practice, various point-of-care testing (POCT) tools are employed, including:

- *Dry hematology:* This technique measures fibrinogen quickly by analyzing how blood flows and resists movement.

- *TEG:* This tool looks at the entire coagulation process, measuring different parameters that reflect how well the blood clots.
- *Thromboelastometry:* Similar to TEG but involves more steps and reagents. It assesses blood clotting but is less direct in measuring fibrinogen.

Customizing care based on individual needs helps mitigate risks and optimize outcomes. Implementing strategies to minimize transfusion reactions involves proper blood component selection, ensuring compatibility, and employing leukoreduction techniques. Adequate pre-transfusion screening and compatibility testing reduce the risk of adverse reactions. Given the risk of iron overload from prolonged transfusions, iron management strategies (e.g., iron chelation therapy) might be considered to mitigate iron-related complications.

SUGGESTED READING

1. Cho MS, Modi P, Sharma S. Transfusion-Related Acute Lung Injury. In: StatPearls [Internet]. Treasure Island (FL): StatPearls Publishing; 2025.
2. Crochemore T, Piza FMT, Rodrigues RDR, Guerra JCC, Ferraz LJR, Corrêa TD. A new era of thromboelastometry. Einstein (Sao Paulo). 2017;15(3):380-5.
3. Escobar MF, Nassar AH, Theron G, Barnea ER, Nicholson W, Ramasauskaite D, et al. FIGO recommendations on the management of postpartum hemorrhage 2022. Int J Gynaecol Obstet. 2022;157 Suppl 1(Suppl 1):3-50.
4. Fredericks C, Kubasiak JC, Mentzer CJ, Yon JR. Massive transfusion: An update for the anesthesiologist. World J Anesthesiol. 2017;6(1):14-21.
5. Fries D. Dilutionskoagulopathie: Entstehung, Diagnostik und Management [Dilutional coagulopathy: development, diagnostic options and management. Hamostaseologie. 2006;26(3 Suppl 1):S15-9.
6. Gehrie EA, Roubinian NH, Chowdhury D, Brambilla DJ, Murphy EL, Gottschall JL, et al.; NHLBI Recipient Epidemiology-Donor Evaluation Study (REDS-III). A multicentre study investigating vital sign changes occurring in complicated and uncomplicated transfusions. Vox Sanguinis. 2018;113(2):160-9.
7. Gerecht R. The lethal triad. Hypothermia, acidosis & coagulopathy create a deadly cycle for trauma patients. JEMS. 2014;39:56-60.
8. Gosmann F, Nørgaard A, Rasmussen MB, Rahbek C, Seeberg J, Møller T. Transfusion-associated circulatory overload in adult, medical emergency patients with perspectives on early warning practice: a single-centre, clinical study. Blood Transfus. 2018;16(2):137-44.
9. Khajavi MR, Etezadi F, Moharari RS, Imani F, Meysamie AP, Khashayar P, et al. Effects of normal saline vs. Lactated ringer's during renal transplantation. Ren Fail. 2008;30(5):535-9.
10. Levy GJ, Shabot MM, Hart ME, Mya WW, Goldfinger D. Transfusion-related noncardiogenic pulmonary edema. Report of a case and a warning regarding treatment. Transfusion. 1986;26:278-81.
11. Moore J, Chandraharan E. Management of massive postpartum haemorrhage and coagulopathy. Obstetr Gynaecol Reprod Med. 2010;20(6):174-80.

12. Mutter TC, Ruth CA, Dart AB. Hydroxyethyl starch (HES) versus other fluid therapies: effects on kidney function. Cochrane Database Syst Rev 2013;7:CD007594.
13. Muñoz M, Stensballe J, Ducloy-Bouthors AS, Bonnet MP, De Robertis E, Fornet I, et al. Patient blood management in obstetrics: prevention and treatment of postpartum haemorrhage. A NATA consensus statement. Blood Transfus. 2019;17(2):112-36.
14. Ngwenya S. Postpartum hemorrhage: incidence, risk factors, and outcomes in a low-resource setting. Int J Women's Health. 22016;8:647-50.
15. Obeagu EI, Obeagu GU. The effects of prolonged term blood transfusion in Postpartum Hemorrhage. Postpartum Hemorrhage. 2024;2:47-58.
16. Owattanapanich N, Chittawatanarat K, Benyakorn T, Sirikun J. Risks and benefits of hypotensive resuscitation in patients with traumatic hemorrhagic shock: a meta-analysis. Scand J Trauma Resusc Emerg Med. 2018;26:107.
17. Prevention and management of postpartum haemorrhage. BJOG. 2016;124: e106-49.
18. Rahim R, Varghese S, Thambi R, Suma MS. Study on acute transfusion related adverse reactions in surgery department. Int J Res Med Sci. 2021;9(5):1381-7.
19. Royal Cornwall Hospitals NHS Trust. (2019). Obstetric Hemorrhage Clinical Guideline V2.3 Royal Cornwall Hospitals NHS Trust. [online] Available from https://doclibrary-rcht.cornwall.nhs.uk/DocumentsLibrary/RoyalCornwallHospitalsTrust/Clinical/MidwiferyAndObstetrics/ObstetricHaemorrhageClinicalGuideline.pdf [Last accessed December, 2025.
20. Shander A, Cappellini MD, Goodnough LT. Iron overload and toxicity: the hidden risk of multiple blood transfusions. Vox Sanguinis. 2009;97(3):185-97.
21. Spahn DR, Bouillon B, Cerny V, Duranteau J, Filipescu D, Hunt BJ, et al. The European guideline on management of major bleeding and coagulopathy following trauma. Crit Care. 2019;23(1):98.
22. Yunos M, Bellomo R, Story D, Kellum J. Bench-to-bedside review: Chloride in critical illness. Crit Care; 2010;14(4):226.

11 CHAPTER

Newer Guidelines in Postpartum Hemorrhage

Kena Gandhi, Manju Puri

INTRODUCTION

Despite ongoing advancements in obstetric care, postpartum hemorrhage (PPH) remains a critical maternal health emergency. In rural settings across India, postpartum hemorrhage remains significantly prevalent, occurring in nearly 12% of all deliveries, with the incidence rising to about 15% in subsequent pregnancies. The 2025 guideline provides a unified, system-based approach emphasizing preparedness, rapid recognition, and timely intervention through structured care bundles. The document highlights the need for strong facility-level systems, multidisciplinary teamwork, and harmonized standards of care.

DEFINITION

Updated Perspective

The guideline moves away from relying only on numerical blood-loss cut-offs, because PPH can occur before reaching high volumes and is often underestimated. Instead, it stresses early action based on clinical condition, speed of bleeding, and physiological deterioration. A blood loss approximately 300 mL accompanied by abnormal vital signs or concerning clinical findings should be considered an early warning sign and treated promptly.

Burden and Risk Factors

Although many antenatal or intrapartum factors are associated with increased bleeding risk, most PPH cases occur unexpectedly. Therefore, every delivery unit must be fully equipped and trained to manage PPH at any time.

PREVENTION OF PPH

Antenatal Strategies

Preventive care begins in pregnancy and includes:

- *Screening for anemia and timely correction:* Where oral iron is poorly tolerated, ineffective, or when rapid correction of iron-deficiency anemia is required, IV iron therapy is recommended over oral supplementation provided that appropriate monitoring for adverse reactions is ensured.

- Ensuring proper antenatal visits and counselling.
- Maintaining sterile practice and evidence-based antimicrobial prophylaxis when required to reduce surgical site infections.

Intrapartum Prevention

Active Management of the Third Stage of Labor

Active management of the third stage of labor (AMTSL) continues to be the most effective universal preventive intervention. Key components include:

- Administration of a uterotonic (preferably oxytocin) after placental delivery
- Delayed cord clamping
- Delivery of placenta by controlled cord traction
- Intermittent fundal assessment

Heat stable carbetocin preferred when cold chain is difficult to maintain.

A large Cochrane review comparing AMTSL with expectant management reported significant benefits with active intervention. Across three studies including 4,636 participants, AMTSL markedly reduced the risk of severe primary PPH (RR 0.34; 95% CI 0.14–0.87; $p = 0.024$). It also lowered the likelihood of postpartum hemoglobin dropping below 9 g/dL, based on evidence from two studies with 1572 women (RR 0.50; 95% CI 0.30–0.83; $p = 0.0076$). In addition, active management was linked to a meaningful decrease in average maternal blood loss and reduced need for additional uterotonic agents when compared with expectant management.

Facility and System-level Preparedness

Prevention also depends on the facility's capacity to respond quickly:

- Consistent availability of uterotonics, tranexamic acid, IV fluids, blood products and essential surgical supplies.
- Updated protocols and context-appropriate operating procedures.
- Regular multidisciplinary emergency drills and simulation.
- Implementation of readiness, recognition, response and learning bundles.

EARLY RECOGNITION OF PPH

The guideline emphasizes that visual estimation is unreliable, and early recognition should focus on combining objective tools with clinical observation.

Identification Bundle

Monitoring should be continuous from pregnancy through postpartum, with structured charts and triggers for escalation.

Physiological Indicators

Essential parameters include:
- Heart rate, blood pressure, respiratory rate.
- Uterine tone assessment.
- Amount and pattern of bleeding.
- General appearance, consciousness, and perfusion signs.

Measurement Tools

Calibrated drapes or containers can be used, but results must always be interpreted alongside clinical judgement and vital signs, as underestimation is common.

MANAGEMENT OF PPH

The 2025 guideline shifts from a step-by-step sequence to a bundled approach, where multiple interventions are initiated simultaneously.

Universal Components

Six elements form the foundation for all PPH cases:
1. *Team activation and leadership:* Quick mobilization of a multi-disciplinary team with clear leadership.
2. *Coordination and communication:* Explicit instructions, closed-loop communication, and timely handovers.
3. *Support to woman and family:* Maintaining dignity, reassurance, and involving the family in decisions.
4. *Readiness and resource access:* Immediate access to critical drugs, equipment, blood, and transport.
5. *Monitoring and documentation:* Frequent assessment of vital signs, ongoing bleeding, and treatment response.
6. *Debrief and quality improvement:* After the event, teams should review the case to identify learning points.

EMOTIVE Bundle Approach

The *EMOTIVE framework*, recommended by the WHO, provides a structured, evidence-based model for PPH management. It outlines a systematic approach designed to improve maternal outcomes. Following the EMOTIVE protocol enables healthcare professionals to deliver timely and effective care.

Early Detection of Blood Loss

Prompt recognition of abnormal bleeding using accurate measurement techniques and close monitoring of maternal clinical signs is essential for timely intervention.

Uterine Massage

Immediate and continuous uterine massage should be performed to enhance uterine contraction. This measure supports bleeding control but must be carried out alongside other definitive treatments.

Uterotonic Medications

Administer uterotonic agents. Most commonly used is oxytocin to stimulate effective uterine contractions. These drugs help minimize blood loss and should be given without delay.

Tranexamic Acid and Intravenous Fluids

Tranexamic acid helps in clot stabilization and reduces ongoing hemorrhage, while IV crystalloids help maintain circulatory stability and adequate tissue perfusion.

Examination and Escalation of Care

Conduct a thorough assessment of the patient's vitals and clinical condition to guide management decisions. Structured escalation protocols ensure timely involvement of senior staff and rapid initiation of advanced interventions when required.

Escalation Interventions

Uterine Balloon Tamponade

The guideline encourages early use of balloon tamponade when bleeding persists despite first-line therapies, especially where surgical support is limited.

Surgical Interventions

If pharmacological measures fail, surgical intervention for PPH should be initiated without delay, preferably within the first golden hour:

- Uterine compression sutures (e.g., B-Lynch).
- Arterial ligation or devascularization techniques.
- Hysterectomy when all other measures fail and the woman's life is at risk.

HEALTH SYSTEM STRENGTHENING

Outcomes depend not only on clinical skill but on system functioning.

Reducing Care Variability

Ensuring uniform quality of care across facilities is critical.

Training

Frequent simulation-based training for obstetric emergencies enhances team performance.

Accountability

Maternal death reviews, morbidity audits, and monitoring guideline adherence are essential for quality improvement.

RESEARCH, INNOVATION, AND IMPLEMENTATION

Areas requiring further study include:

- More precise physiological thresholds to aid early recognition.
- Evaluation of implementation strategies for clinical bundles.
- Development of newer uterotonic options.
- Improved detection tools for coagulopathy at point-of-care.

Implementation research will be central in translating these guidelines into practice across diverse health systems.

CONCLUSION

The 2025 PPH guideline marks a significant shift toward earlier recognition, combined interventions, and strengthened systems of care. Consistent application of these updated strategies across all maternity settings can substantially reduce preventable maternal deaths and complications.

KEY TAKE-HOME MESSAGES

- PPH continues to be a major cause of maternal mortality worldwide.
- The latest guideline prioritizes physiological signs and clinical deterioration rather than fixed blood-loss thresholds.
- Prevention relies on AMTSL, correction of antenatal anemia, and strong facility-level readiness.
- Early diagnosis requires structured monitoring, objective tools, and continuous vigilance.
- Management emphasizes initiating multiple interventions simultaneously, including uterotonics, TXA, fluids, balloon tamponade and timely surgical escalation.
- Effective team communication, leadership, and respectful care form universal components of PPH management.
- Successful implementation depends on adequate resources, training and quality-assurance systems.
- Standardized bundles help reduce differences in care quality between facilities.

SUGGESTED READING

1. Escobar MF, Nassar AH, Theron G, Barnea ER, Nicholson W, Ramasauskaite D, et al. FIGO recommendations on the management of postpartum haemorrhage 2022. Int J Gynecol Obstet. 2022;157(Suppl. 1):3-50.

2. Evensen A, Anderson JM, Fontaina P. Postpartum haemorrhage: prevention and treatment. Am Fam Physician. 2017;95(7):442-9.
3. Geller SE, Goudar SS, Adams MG, Naik VA, Patel A, Bellad MB, et al. Factors associated with acute postpartum hemorrhage in low-risk women delivering in rural India. Int J Gynaecol Obstet. 2008;101(1):94-9.
4. Nicholson L, Axon E, Daru J, Rogozińska E. Effect and safety of intravenous iron compared with oral iron for treatment of iron-deficiency anaemia in pregnancy. Cochrane Database Syst Rev. 2024;12(12):CD016136.
5. World Health Organization. Consolidated guidelines for the prevention, diagnosis and treatment of postpartum haemorrhage. Genva: World Health Organization; 2025.
6. World Health Organization. WHO guideline on haemoglobin cut offs and management of anaemia in pregnancy. Geneva: WHO; 2023.
7. World Health Organization. WHO recommendations: Uterotonics for the prevention of postpartum haemorrhage. Geneva: WHO; 2022.

12 CHAPTER

Newer Modalities in Postpartum Hemorrhage

Deepti Gupta, Shuchi Sehgal

INTRODUCTION

Postpartum hemorrhage (PPH) remains a devastating obstetric emergency and the leading cause of maternal mortality worldwide, accounting for approximately 27% of maternal deaths globally and affecting approximately 12% women in India. Defined as cumulative blood loss ≥1,000 mL or blood loss accompanied by hypovolemia signs within 24 hours of delivery, PPH challenges clinicians with its unpredictable nature—up to 40% of cases occur in women without identifiable risk factors. The traditional "4 T's" framework (Tone, Trauma, Tissue, and Thrombin) continues to guide management, but recent technological and pharmacological innovations are transforming our approach.

Management of PPH revolves around four major components which need to be executed simultaneously-communication, resuscitation, monitoring investigation and arrest of bleeding. Furthermore therapeutic goals include- maintaining hemoglobin >8 g/dL, platelet count >75 × 10^9/L, prothrombin <1.5 × mean control, activated prothrombin time <1.5 × mean control, fibrinogen >1.0 g/L. This chapter examines advances in PPH management that promise to significantly reduce maternal morbidity and mortality through enhanced prevention, rapid diagnosis, and targeted interventions.

PHARMACOLOGICAL REVOLUTION: BEYOND OXYTOCIN

Uterotonic Innovations

The pharmacological armamentarium for uterine atony (responsible for 70–80% of PPH cases) has expanded beyond traditional agents like oxytocin and ergometrine. Novel formulations and delivery systems are optimizing efficacy while minimizing side effects:

- *Heat-stable carbetocin:* This long-acting oxytocin analog represents a breakthrough in tropical settings where cold-chain storage is unreliable. Carbetocin is a long-acting synthetic analogue of oxytocin with half-life of 40 minutes. Following IV administration, onset of contraction is seen in 2 minutes with sustained and rhythmic contractions for 6 and 60 minutes respectively. Following intramuscular administration, sustained and rhythmic contractions last for 11 and 120 minutes, respectively. It can be stored at temperatures up to 30°C. single-dose administration provides sustained uterine protection comparable to multiple-dose oxytocin regimens. According to Cochrane review, There is evidence to show the benefit of carbetocin over oxytocin for preventing PPH following cesarean deliveries. Carbetocin should also be considered as an option over syntometrine, due to the lower likelihood of adverse effects. The World Health Organization recommends heat-stable carbetocin for PPH prevention in resource-limited settings, where it demonstrates superior cost-effectiveness despite higher initial costs.

- *Intrauterine instillation:* Research demonstrates that direct intrauterine administration of diluted oxytocin (via intrauterine catheters) achieves 10-fold higher myometrial concentrations compared to intravenous routes. This targeted approach may revolutionize refractory atony management, especially in high-risk patients.

Hemostatic Adjuncts

- *Tranexamic acid (TXA):* The landmark WOMAN trial established TXA as a life-saving intervention when administered within three hours of delivery. New protocols emphasize point-of-care availability and weight-based dosing (1 g IV repeated if ongoing bleeding). Emerging evidence suggests that pre-emptive administration during cesarean delivery for high-risk patients reduces blood loss by 30–40% without increasing thrombotic complications.
- *Fibrinogen concentrate:* Research reveals that fibrinogen depletion (<2 g/L) occurs earlier than previously recognized in PPH and strongly predicts severity. Unlike fresh frozen plasma (requiring thawing and cross-matching), lyophilized fibrinogen concentrate enables rapid, targeted repletion. The FIDEL trial demonstrated that early and systematic administration of 3 g fibrinogen concentrate did not reduce blood loss, transfusion needs or postpartum anemia, but did prevent plasma fibrinogen decrease without any subsequent thromboembolic events.
  Novel pharmacological agents in PPH management is shown in **Table 1**.

Minimally Invasive and Mechanical Innovations

Advanced Tamponade Systems

Uterine balloon tamponade (UBT) has evolved from improvised solutions to sophisticated devices with enhanced efficacy:

- *Pressure-controlled balloons:* It was the first uterine tamponade balloon system designed specifically for the treatment of obstetric hemorrhage. It consists of a silicone balloon (maximum recommended fill volume 500 mL), connected to a 24 French silicone catheter 54 cm in length.

TABLE 1: Novel pharmacological agents in PPH management.

Agent	*Mechanism*	*Advantages*	*Evidence level*
Heat-stable carbetocin	Long-acting oxytocin receptor agonist	Single-dose, thermostable, 60–90 min half-life	WHO recommendation (Phase III trials)
Nanoemulsified TXA	Enhanced antifibrinolytic delivery	Rapid sublingual absorption, no IV access needed	Phase II trials
Polidocanol foam	Sclerosant for persistent oozing	Topical application, minimally invasive	Multicenter prospective studies
Fibrinogen concentrate	Targeted coagulation factor replacement	Rapid administration, no cross-match needed	FIDEL trial (RCT)

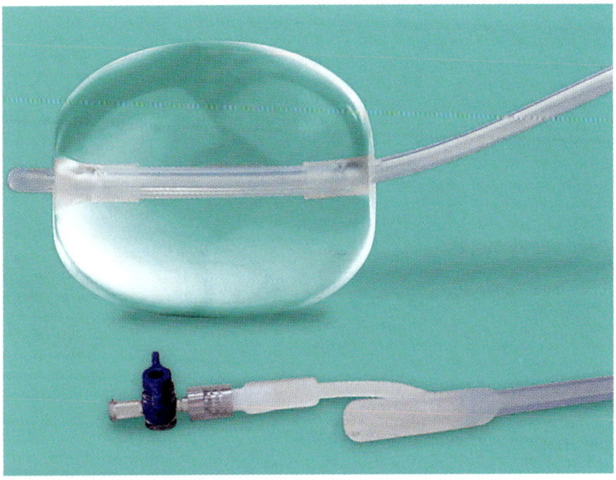

Fig. 1: Bakri balloon.

Devices like the Bakri SOS Balloon now incorporate integrated pressure sensors and automated infusion systems (BakriOne) that maintain optimal intrauterine pressure (typically 70–80 mm Hg). This prevents under-distension (ineffective tamponade) and over-distension (tissue necrosis risk). Recent modifications include concomitant intrauterine irrigation channels that permit continuous blood loss monitoring. **Figure 1** showing Bakri Balloon.

- *BT-Cath*—the BT-Cath is a silicone balloon (maximum recommended fill volume 500 mL) with an inverted pear shape to conform to the shape of the uterine cavity. **Figure 2** showing BT Cath balloon
- *EBB tamponade system:* The ebb tamponade system is a dual polyurethane balloon device containing an upper uterine balloon

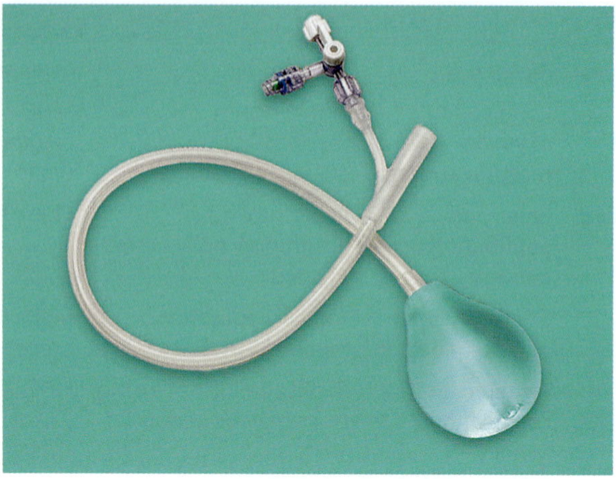

Fig. 2: BT-Cath.

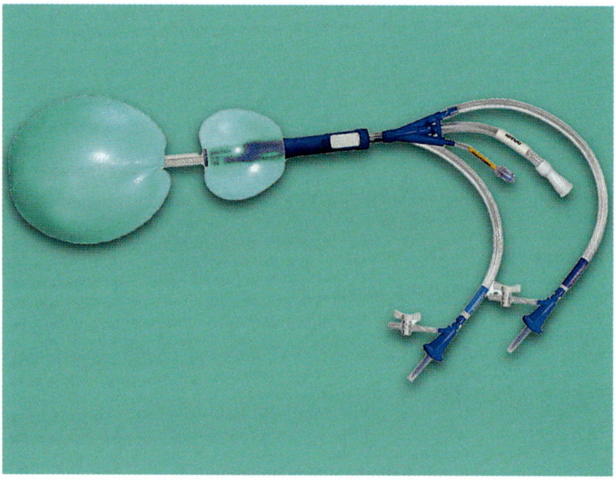

Fig. 3: EBB tamponade system.

(maximum recommended fill volume 750 mL) and a lower vaginal balloon (maximum recommended fill volume 300 mL). A central drain allows for monitoring of possible ongoing or recurrent hemorrhage from above the uterine balloon. **Figure 3** showing EBB tamponade system.

- *Condom catheter tamponade:* In resource-limited settings, low-cost alternatives demonstrate remarkable efficacy. CG Balloon overcomes the major disadvantages of conventional condom balloon tamponade by having a drainage channel for assessing the uterine bleeding. It uses rings cut out of catheter only and not the thread to tie the condom to catheter which avoids loose/too tight knots as well as infection, saves time and is simple to use. CG Balloon is successful in 92.3% cases as a

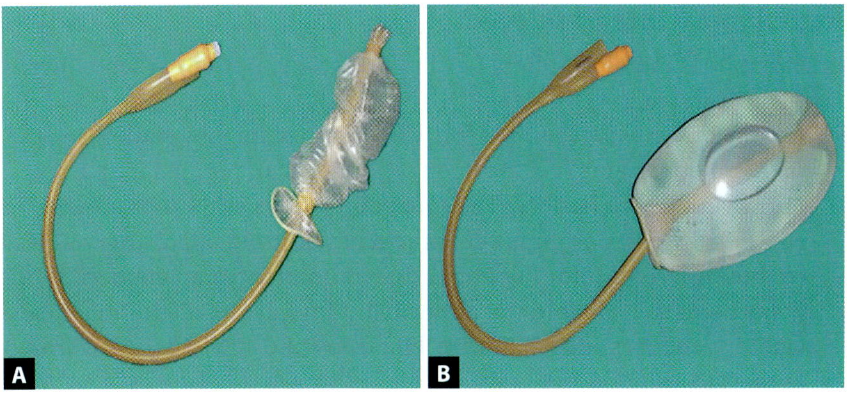

Figs. 4A and B: Condom catheter tamponade.

second-line approach in atonic PPH protocols when first-line treatment fails and before more costly and risky surgery. It can also be used for extended indications for lower genital tract tears or placental bed oozing as it allows the drainage of uterine bleeding simultaneously **(Figs. 4A and B)**.

Nonpneumatic Antishock Garment

It is a low technology first-aid device that buys a woman time to seek definitive and adequate treatment. Made of neoprene and Velcro (Velcro Industries), the non-pneumatic anti-shock garment (NASG) comprises six segments: an ankle segment pair, a calf segment pair, a thigh segment pair, a pelvic segment, and two abdominal segments. Its advantages are manyfold including:

- Circumferential counter-pressure decreases blood flow to the lower body while increasing circulation in the vital organs of the upper body.
- Serves to reverse shock and provide time for transportation, blood transfusion, or surgery, particularly in under-resourced and overcrowded settings.
- Designed to provide total perineal access as well as stretching in the abdominal segment so that the condition of the uterus can be assessed.
- NASG application improves access to veins in the arm, thus aiding fluid replacement.
- Can be safely worn for up to 48 hours, may help avoid unnecessary emergency hysterectomy for intractable uterine atony, and may decrease the need for or the number of blood transfusions.
- Reusable and can be disinfected with a 0.01% bleach solution, laundered, hung to dry, and has been tested to last at least 72 washings/uses.

Radiological Interventions

Interventional radiology offers fertility-preserving options when conventional measures fail:

- *Uterine artery embolization (UAE):* Modern techniques employ temporary embolic agents (gelatin sponge) rather than permanent particles, preserving future fertility. The procedure achieves 85–92% success in controlled studies, with newer approaches utilizing radial artery access (reducing groin complications) and outpatient management. UAE is particularly valuable for abnormally invasive placentation cases, where it reduces intraoperative blood loss by 40% when performed prophylactically.
- *Pre-operative prophylactic balloon artery occlusion (PBAO):* For known placenta accreta spectrum disorders, pre-cesarean placement of internal iliac or common femoral artery balloons enables immediate inflation during delivery. Contemporary protocols emphasize partial inflation rather than complete occlusion, balancing hemorrhage control against ischemic risks.

Point-of-Care Diagnostics and Monitoring

Viscoelastic Hemostatic Assays

Traditional coagulation tests (PT, aPTT, fibrinogen) have 30–60 minute turnaround times—prohibitive in active hemorrhage. Rotational thromboelastometry (ROTEM®) and thromboelastography (TEG®) provide real-time, comprehensive coagulation profiles at the bedside within 10–15 minutes:

- *FIBTEM assay:* Specifically measures functional fibrinogen, identifying depletion earlier than conventional tests. Studies demonstrate that FIBTEM A5 <12 mm predicts severe PPH progression with 92% sensitivity.
- *Goal-directed transfusion:* Viscoelastic hemostatic assay (VHA)-guided algorithms reduce blood product wastage and transfusion-associated complications. The OBS2 trial showed a 35% reduction in FFP and platelet transfusions using ROTEM-guided protocols compared to fixed-ratio resuscitation.

Quantitative Blood Loss Revolution

Visual estimation notoriously underestimates blood loss by 30–50%. Modern quantitative blood loss (QBL) systems integrate multiple modalities:

- *Gravimetric measurement:* Automated systems calculate blood loss by weight differences of soaked materials, validated against artificial intelligence (AI) algorithms.
- *Colorimetric drapes:* Calibrated under-buttock drapes provide instant visual quantification through distinct color zones.

- *Mobile applications:* AI-enabled apps (e.g., Triton®) use computer vision technology to analyze suction canister images, providing real-time loss estimates.

Ultrasound Innovations

Portable ultrasound extends beyond FAST exams in PPH:

- *Uterine contractility assessment:* 3-D volumetric ultrasound objectively evaluates myometrial contraction strength, differentiating atony from retained tissue.
- *Vascular mapping:* Doppler identifies arteriovenous malformations or pseudoaneurysms requiring targeted intervention.
- *Resuscitation guidance:* Inferior vena cava (IVC) collapsibility index >50% predicts fluid responsiveness better than blood pressure in compensated shock.

Surgical and System-based Advances

Refined Surgical Techniques

Novel approaches minimize morbidity while maximizing efficacy:

- *Stepwise uterine devascularization:* The new FIGO protocol advocates systematic ligation sequence: uterine → utero-ovarian anastomoses → internal iliac arteries. This achieves 90% hemostasis while preserving ovarian function.
- *Compression sutures:* Modified techniques like the "Nieto-Calcified Square Suture" incorporate vertical transverse compression with reduced synechiae risk compared to B-Lynch sutures.
- *Selective embolization:* Combining intraoperative ultrasound with absorbable gelatin pledgets enables targeted vessel occlusion without radiology suite transfer.

Comprehensive Hemorrhage Protocols (Fig. 5)

Comprehensive Hemorrhage Protocols are shown in **Figure 5**.

FUTURE DIRECTIONS AND CONCLUSION

Emerging Frontiers

Several promising technologies approach clinical implementation:

- *Endo-uterine vacuum-induced devices:* The Jada® System applies controlled negative pressure (–80 mm Hg) directly to the endometrial surface, stimulating myometrial contraction and apposing raw surfaces. Early trials demonstrate 94% efficacy for atony refractory to first-line uterotonics.
- *Resuscitative endovascular balloon occlusion (REBOA):* Adapted from trauma surgery, zone III REBOA (infrarenal aortic occlusion) stabilizes

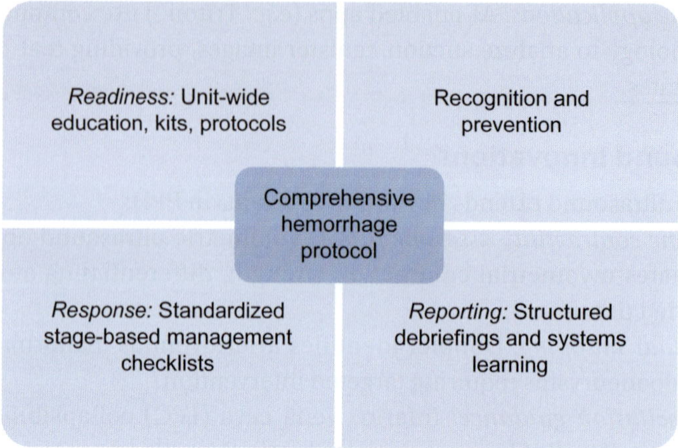

Fig. 5: Comprehensive hemorrhage protocols.

patients in extremis during transfer to definitive care. Newer partial flow catheters mitigate ischemic risks during prolonged use.

- *Topical hemostatic agents:* Fibrin spray patches and gelatin-thrombin matrices show promise for diffuse oozing from placental beds, particularly in coagulopathic patients.

IMPLEMENTATION CHALLENGES AND EQUITY

Despite these advances, disparities in PPH outcomes persist globally. High-income countries report mortality rates <0.02%, while low-resource settings face rates 100-fold higher. Bridging this gap requires:

- *Affordable innovations:* Scaling production of condom tamponade kits and heat-stable carbetocin.
- *Task-sharing models:* Training non-physician providers in balloon tamponade and TXA administration.
- *Digital health integration:* mHealth applications guiding community health workers through PPH algorithms.

CONCLUSION

The landscape of PPH management has transformed dramatically, shifting from reactive, procedure-heavy approaches to proactive, precision-based strategies. By integrating advanced diagnostics (viscoelastic testing, ultrasound), targeted therapeutics (fibrinogen concentrate, TXA), and minimally invasive interventions (embolization, vacuum devices), clinicians can now address hemorrhage with unprecedented precision. However, technology alone cannot eliminate PPH mortality—success requires standardized protocols, interdisciplinary coordination, and equitable implementation. As these innovations permeate global practice, the vision of eliminating preventable maternal death from hemorrhage moves steadily toward realization. Continued research into prediction algorithms, novel hemostatics, and system-level interventions remains crucial to achieving this goal.

SUGGESTED READING

1. Anderson JM, Etches D. Prevention and management of postpartum hemorrhage. Am Fam Physician. 2007;75(6):875-82.
2. Bakri Y, B-Lynch C, Alouini S. Second generation of intrauterine balloon tamponade: new perspective. BMJ Innov. 2020 Jan;6(1):1-3.
3. Cho SB, Hong SJ, Lee S, Won JH, Choi HC, Ha JY, et al. Preoperative Prophylactic Balloon-Assisted Occlusion of the Internal Iliac Arteries in the Management of Placenta Increta/Percreta. Medicina (Kaunas). 2020;56(8):368.
4. Ducloy-Bouthors AS, Mercier FJ, Grouin JM, Bayoumeu F, Corouge J, Le Gouez A, et al; FIDEL working group. Early and systematic administration of fibrinogen concentrate in postpartum haemorrhage following vaginal delivery: the FIDEL randomised controlled trial. BJOG. 2021;128(11):1814-23.
5. FIGO Safe Motherhood and Newborn Health Committee. Non-pneumatic anti-shock garment to stabilize women with hypovolemic shock secondary to obstetric hemorrhage. International J Gynecol Obstetr. 2015;128:194-5.
6. Hunter DJ, Schulz P, Wassenaar W. Effect of carbetocin, a long-acting oxytocin analog on the postpartum uterus. Clin Pharmacol Ther. 1992;52:60-7.
7. Mishra N, Agrawal S, Gulabani K, Shrivastava C. Use of an Innovative Condom Balloon Tamponade in Postpartum Haemorrhage: A Report. J Obstet Gynaecol India. 2016;66(1):63-7.
8. Patel, M. Postpartum Hemorrhage: Enhancing Outcomes for Mothers by Effective Management. J Obstet Gynecol India. 2024;74:191-5.
9. Quantitative Blood Loss in Obstetric Hemorrhage: ACOG COMMITTEE OPINION, Number 794. Obstet Gynecol. 2019;134(6):e150-6.
10. Shakur H, Elbourne D, Gülmezoglu M, Alfirevic Z, Ronsmans C, Allen E, Roberts I. The WOMAN Trial (World Maternal Antifibrinolytic Trial): tranexamic acid for the treatment of postpartum haemorrhage: an international randomised, double blind placebo controlled trial. Trials. 2010;11:40.
11. Stainsby D, MacLennan S, Thomas D, Isaac J, Hamilton PJ. Guidelines on the management of massive blood loss. Br J Haematol. 2006;135:634-41.
12. Su LL, Chong YS, Samuel M. Carbetocin for preventing postpartum haemorrhage. Cochrane Database Syst Rev. 2012;2012(4):CD005457.
13. WOMAN Trial Collaborators. Effect of early tranexamic acid administration on mortality, hysterectomy, and other morbidities in women with postpartum haemorrhage (WOMAN): an international, randomised, double-blind, placebo-controlled trial. Lancet. 2017;389(10084):2105-16.

13 CHAPTER

Bundle Approach—E-MOTIVE

Poorva Badkur, Nitu Mishra

"A mother's life is in our hands; our knowledge, preparedness, and swift action make the difference between life and loss."

—Unknown

INTRODUCTION

A significant decline in maternal mortality was accomplished during the Millennium Development Goal (MDG) period from 2000 to 2015. The global Maternal Mortality Ratio (MMR) was 227 deaths per 100,000 live births in 2015. However, progress has slowed recently, with the global MMR declining to only 223 deaths per 100,000 live births in 2020. A similar trend is evident in India, showcasing remarkable progress in lowering its MMR between 2000 (MMR-384) and 2015 (MMR-130), but a staggered progress to MMR of 97 deaths per 100,000 live births in 2020. An estimated 287,000 women globally lost their lives due to maternal causes in 2020. This alarming figure translates to nearly 800 deaths every day—or one maternal death every two minutes. Sub-Saharan Africa and Asia account for 85% of global maternal deaths. Postpartum hemorrhage (PPH) remains a leading cause of maternal mortality in India. Over time, the World Health Organization (WHO) and other regulatory bodies have provided guidelines for the prevention of PPH; despite the guidelines, the deaths due to PPH remain high. Central to the challenge in PPH is the delay in the diagnosis of PPH, which ultimately leads to a delay in treatment.

BUNDLE CARE APPROACH

In 2001, the Institute for Healthcare Improvement (IHI) introduced a structured approach to care bundling to enhance the quality and efficiency of healthcare delivery. This method involves implementing small sets of evidence-based interventions together, producing significantly better outcomes than applying them individually.

In 2012, WHO published its "Recommendations for the Prevention and Treatment of Postpartum Hemorrhage" to provide evidence-informed clinical care recommendations for hemorrhage due to uterine atony. However, adherence to these recommendations remains a challenge. The bundle approach has been proposed as a potential solution to suboptimal adherence to PPH guidelines. In early 2017, WHO decided to explore whether bundling current WHO-recommended evidenced-based interventions for PPH due to uterine atony might accelerate adoption and adherence to PPH guidelines.

Three PPH care bundles were initially identified as meeting the agreed criteria: (1) prevention and recognition of PPH, (2) first response to PPH, and (3) response to refractory PPH. The prevention and recognition of the PPH bundle approach closely resembles the Active Management of the Third Stage of Labor (AMTSL) package, which the WHO has de-emphasized in recent years as a care strategy. So, the first one was rejected out of these three care bundles, and the other two were accepted.

The objective of PPH Emergency care using a bundle approach is to enhance the quality of care at delivery facilities. It involves addressing both *clinical* and *non-clinical* aspects, each playing a vital role in improving outcomes. Clinical elements focus on evidence-based interventions, timely management, and skilled healthcare providers, while non-clinical aspects emphasize teamwork, communication, facility readiness, and leadership. Together, these components ensure a comprehensive and effective response to PPH emergencies.

The set of interventions in the first response PPH bundle and refractory PPH bundle response is enumerated in **Box 1**.

The first response bundle meets the characteristics and criteria for the bundle approach defined by the IHI. It comprises four universally recommended interventions, which are to be administered without exception to all women experiencing PPH caused by uterine atony. But the refractory PPH response bundle was designed to manage critically ill women who continued to bleed despite initial measures, with their condition worsening

BOX 1: Final care bundles for postpartum hemorrhage.

First response PPH bundle:
- Uterotonic drugs
- Isotonic crystalloids
- Tranexamic acid
- Uterine massage

Notes: Initial fluid resuscitation is performed together with intravenous (IV) administration of uterotonics. If IV uterotonics are not available, fluid resuscitation should be started in parallel with sublingual misoprostol or other parenteral uterotonics. If postpartum hemorrhage (PPH) is in the context of placental retention, the placenta should be extracted and a single dose of antibiotics should be administered.

Response to refractory PPH bundle:
- Compressive measure (aortic compression or bimanual uterine compression)
- Intrauterine balloon tamponade
- Nonpneumatic anti shock garment

Notes: A continuing dose of uterotonics (e.g., oxytocin diluted in isotonic crystalloids) and a second dose of tranexamic acid should be administered during the application of this bundle

or deteriorating. However, this narrow definition might create uncertainties for clinicians when treating women with refractory PPH whose condition remains initially stable.

EMOTIVE

Despite the introduction of Bundle approach in PPH management, there was increasing concern about the delayed recognition of PPH onset. In this context of poor diagnosis of PPH, delayed treatment, and inconsistent use of recommended interventions, WHO convened a group of over 130 stakeholders for the first Global Summit on Postpartum Hemorrhage (PPH Summit) in March 2023. It was concluded that the facilities in LMICs currently rely on visual estimation of blood loss, which is widely recognized as inaccurate and can result in underestimation and hence delayed and low usage of WHO PPH first response bundle.

In December 2023 the WHO released the new guideline combining assessment of postpartum blood loss by calibrated drape and use the treatment bundle of WHO 2017 guideline—The E-MOTIVE for managing postpartum hemorrhage.

The acronym E-MOTIVE stands for:

- E—Early detection of PPH using a calibrated drape.

It is followed rapidly by (in no particular order):

- M—Massage of the uterus
- O—Administration of an oxytocic
- T—Administration of tranexamic acid
- IV—Administration of intravenous fluids
- E—Examination for, identifying and managing the source of bleeding and escalation to more advanced care if bleeding persists

The use of the E-MOTIVE treatment bundle in the management of PPH has been incorporated into the new WHO guidelines on PPH management.

This 2023 guidelines have two key recommendations:

1. Routine objective assessment of postpartum blood loss with a calibrated drape to improve the detection and treatment of PPH.
2. Standardised and timely treatment approach to PPH management through objective blood loss assessment and use of a treatment bundle.

Additional considerations include:

- The recommendation is basically for vaginal delivery.
- The individual interventions should be used for caesarean section as applicable.
- The interventions should ideally be initiated within 15 minutes of diagnosis of PPH.
- Where a woman continues to bleed after receiving all interventions within the PPH treatment bundle, there should be a prompt referral to

a higher-level healthcare facility or a senior clinical provider capable of providing further management.

CONCLUSION

The development and implementation of care bundles should not hinder healthcare providers from thoroughly assessing the underlying cause of PPH before initiating interventions. Accurate identification of the etiology is essential for tailoring the appropriate treatment. Strengthening early detection protocols, improving provider training, and ensuring adherence to care bundles are critical steps to address these challenges effectively.

Relying solely on the passive dissemination of new clinical guidelines, including care bundles, is generally insufficient to achieve sustained behavior changes and enhancements in the quality of care. Active strategies, such as training, hands-on implementation support, and regular feedback, are critical for ensuring these guidelines are effectively adopted and consistently applied.

SUGGESTED READING

1. Althabe F, Therrien MNS, Pingray V, Hermida J, Gülmezoglu AM, Armbruster D, et al. Postpartum hemorrhage care bundles to improve adherence to guidelines: A WHO technical consultation. Int J Gynecol Obstet. 2019;148(3):290-9.
2. FOGSI. (2022). PPH Prevention and Management: Updated PPH Guidelines. [online] Available from https://www.fogsi.org/wp-content/uploads/tog/pph-prevention-and-management-updated-sept-2022.pdf [Last accessed December, 2025].
3. Gallos I, Devall A, Martin J, Middleton L, Beeson L, Galadanci H, et al. Randomized trial of early detection and treatment of postpartum hemorrhage. N Engl J Med. 2023;389(1):11-21.
4. Ministry of Health and Family Welfare. (2022). National health family survey. [online] Available from https://www.pib.gov.in/PressReleasePage.aspx?PRID=1805731 [Last accessed December, 2025].
5. Resar R, Griffin FA, Haraden C, Nolan TW. Using Care Bundles to Improve Health Care Quality. IHI Innovation Series white paper. Cambridge, MA: Institute for Healthcare Improvement; 2012.
6. World Health Organization. WHO Recommendations for the Prevention and Treatment of Postpartum Haemorrhage. Geneva: World Health Organization; 2012.
7. World Health Organization. WHO recommendations on the assessment of postpartum blood loss and use of a treatment bundle for postpartum haemorrhage. Geneva: WHO; 2023.
8. World Health Organization. World health statistics 2020: monitoring health for the SDGs: sustainable development goals. Geneva, Switzerland: World Health Organization; 2020.
9. World Health Organization. (2023). A roadmap to combat postpartum haemorrhage between 2023 and 2030. [online] Available from https://cdn.who.int/media/docs/default-source/reproductive-health/maternal-health/pph-roadmap.pdf [Last accessed December, 2025].

14 CHAPTER

Golden Hour Postpartum Hemorrhage

Kiran Chandna

INTRODUCTION

Golden hour for management of PPH is crucial concept in obstetric care.

The golden hour in PPH is initial 60 minutes following delivery during which prompt recognition and intervention can significantly impact the outcome.

MAIN OBJECTIVE

- *Early recognition* of early signs of PPH and identify the risk factors:
  - Blood loss is <20%—patient is anxious, sweating cold extremities
  - Blood loss from 20–40%—additional tachycardia, tachypnoea, postural hypotension, and oliguria
  - Blood loss >40%—additional hypotension and confusion
- *Assessment:* Evaluate the amount of blood loss and maternal hemodynamics.
- *Stabilization*—administration of uterotonics, fluid resuscitation and blood transfusion
- *Intervention*—perform uterine message, bimanual compression and surgical intervention

GOLDEN HOUR INTERVENTION

- *Uterotonics*—administer oxytocin, methylergometrine, carbetocin prostodin within 1–2 minutes
- *Fluid resuscitation*—provide crystalloid or colloid solution with wide bore cannula to maintain blood pressure and perfusion within 5–10 minute
- *Blood transfusion*—administer blood products packed RBC, FPP, Platelet to correct anemia and coagulopathy within 30–60 minutes
- *Uterine tamponade*—use balloon tamponade/uterine packing to control bleeding within 30–60 minutes

GOLDEN HOUR MONITORING

- *Vital signs*—continuous monitoring of maternal blood pressure, pulse, oxygen saturation and respiratory rate

Calculate shock index and modified shock index

- *Uterine tone*—assess the uterine tone and contraction
- *Bleeding*—do the quantitative assessment of blood loss. By Visual assessment—blood loss is usually underestimated
- *Lab tests*—hemoglobin, coagulation profile to guide management

GOLDEN HOUR TEAM WORK

Call for Help

- Multidisciplinary team work with obstetrician, anesthetist, nurse and other paramedical staff professional with PPH management
- Clear communication—ensure clear communication amongst members to facilitate prompt decision making,
- Standardized protocols-establish standardized protocols for PPH management to ensure consistency and efficiency

IMPORTANCE OF GOLDEN HOUR

By prompt recognition, assessment, and intervention in golden hour, HCP can significantly reduce risk of maternal mortality and morbidity associated with PPH. The golden hour emphasizes the importance of timely and effective care to ensure patient safety.

CHALLENGES AND SOLUTIONS

- *Delayed recognition:* Implement standardized protocols for PPH recognition and response
- Inadequate staffing—ensure adequate staffing and training with PPH drills
- Limited resources
- Communication gap
- Lack of standardized PPH protocols

CONSEQUENCE OF MISSING THE GOLDEN HOUR

Maternal

- Increased risk of mortality due to severe bleeding, hypotension shock and organ failure
- Severe maternal morbidity, prolonged hospital stay and ICU admission
- Coagulopathy and transfusion related complication like TRALI (transfusion related acute lung injury)
- Organ dysfunction-prolonged hypotension and hypoxia can lead to acute kidney damage, liver failure, respiratory failure

Healthcare

- Prolonged hospital stay, increased cost, ICU admissions, patient dissatisfaction, medicolegal implications, reputation damage
- Anxiety for healthcare person and family

PREVENTIVE STRATEGIES

- Standardized PPH protocols for early recognition, assessment and intervention
- Regular training and education by mock drills
- Ensure access to blood bank and timely arrangement of blood products
- Prevention by risk assessment, AMTSL, vigilant care specially in first hour after delivery
- Recognition at earliest by clinical signs and bleeding assessment (visual and quantitative), uterine tone and local examination
- Early response within 5 minutes

STABILIZATION AND INTERVENTION BY BUNDLE APPROACH

Stabilization: Administer uterotonic agents, fluid resuscitation and blood transfusion

Intervention: Perform uterine message, bimanual compression, surgical intervention like repair laceration or tear in vagina or cervix, uterine compression stitches B-Lynch, step wise devascularization, internal iliac artery ligation, embolization or subtotal hysterectomy

Every minute in golden hour is precious.

Golden Hour Timeline

- *0–5 minutes*—recognize the risk factor and sign of bleeding PV
- *5–15 minutes*—assess the severity of bleeding and maternal vitals PR, BP, RR, shock index, modified shock index
- *15–30 minutes*—uterotonics and fluid resuscitation
- *30–60 minutes—continue stabilization and intervention*

Importance of Golden Hour in PPH

Early recognition and prompt intervention can reduce maternal morbidity and mortality. Prompt management will enhance patient safety and improved outcome.

If we miss the golden hour:

- Severe complication in form of maternal mortality
- Delayed recognition and management will lead to massive hemorrhage, shock, organ failure

- Prolonged hospitalization, ICU admissions, long term health problems
- Coagulopathy, transfusion-related complications of massive transfusion and TRALI (transfusion-related acute lung injury)
- Organ dysfunction due to prolonged hypotension (acute kidney injury, respiratory failure)
- Prolonged admission and increase healthcare cost
- Delayed recognition and intervention results in adverse outcomes and medicolegal implications

Preventive Strategies

- Implement standardized protocols for PPH recognition, assessment and intervention
- Regular training of staff for early recognition and rapid action to inform team
- Timely access to blood products (packed RBC, FFP, and platelet)
- Active management of third stage of labor **(Fig. 1)**
- Careful monitoring of patient during post-delivery or post-operative period
- Often the attendants are busy with neonate and celebrating and staff can ignore the patient due to tiredness
- Better to keep patient in labor recovery room for first two hours and do close monitoring of vitals and blood loss
- Correct estimation of blood loss is essential

PROMPT ACTION

- Act promptly under such situations **(Fig. 2)**
- Always call for help as team work will give better prognosis and management

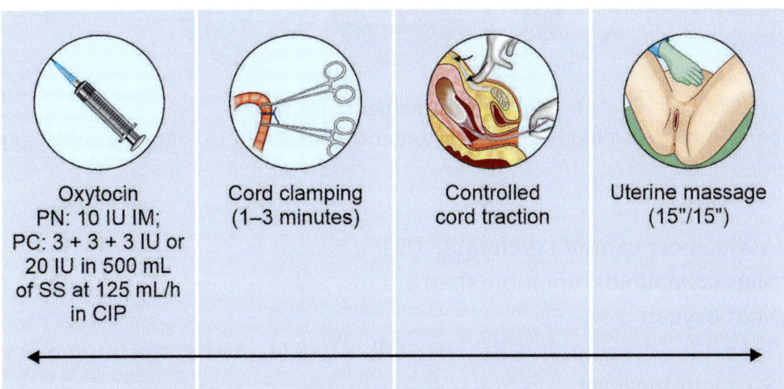

Fig. 1: Active management of the third period of delivery.

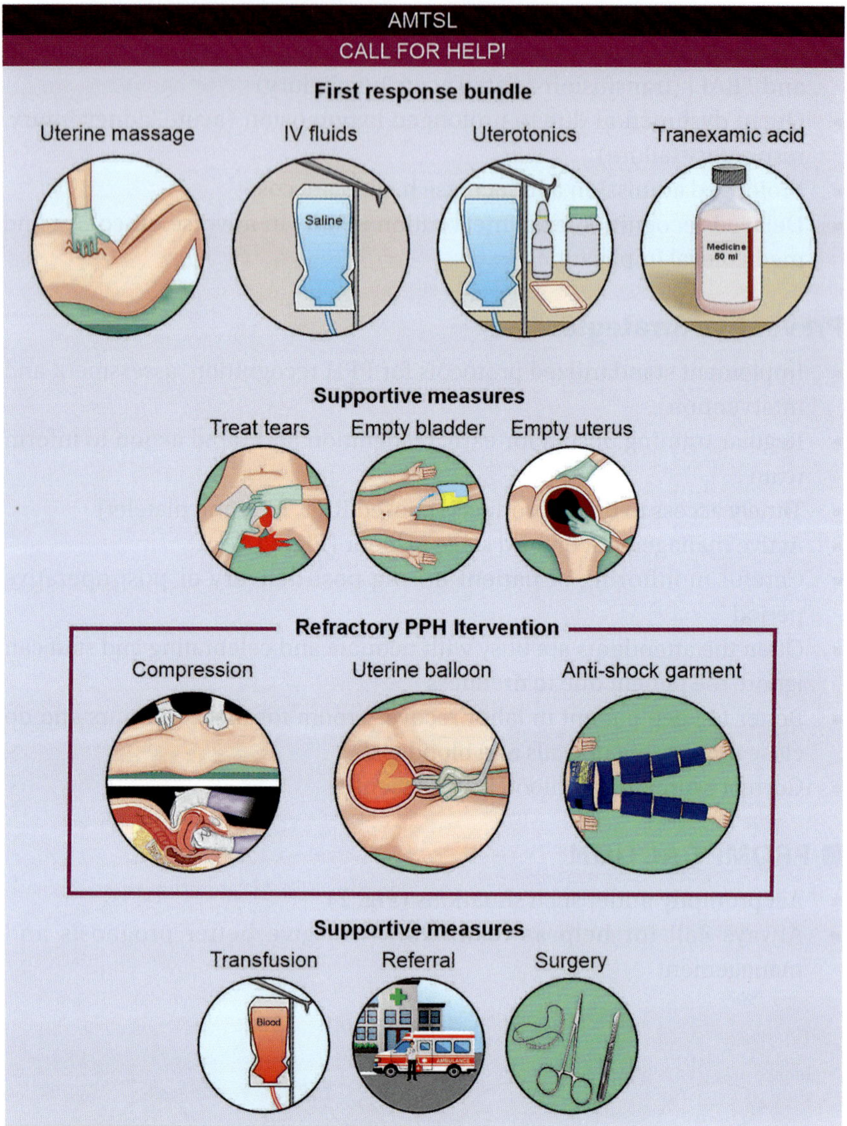

Fig. 2: PPH emergency response.
Source: https://savemothers.org/wp-content/uploads/2021/07/bundle-card-2.jpg.

- A wide bore cannula preferably 16G
- Start crystalloids, not more than 2 L
- Start oxygen
- Take blood samples CBC, BT, CT, PT, PTI, APTT, fibrinogen level, S. Creatinine level
- Remember 4 T as cause for PPH (tone, trauma, tissue, thrombin)

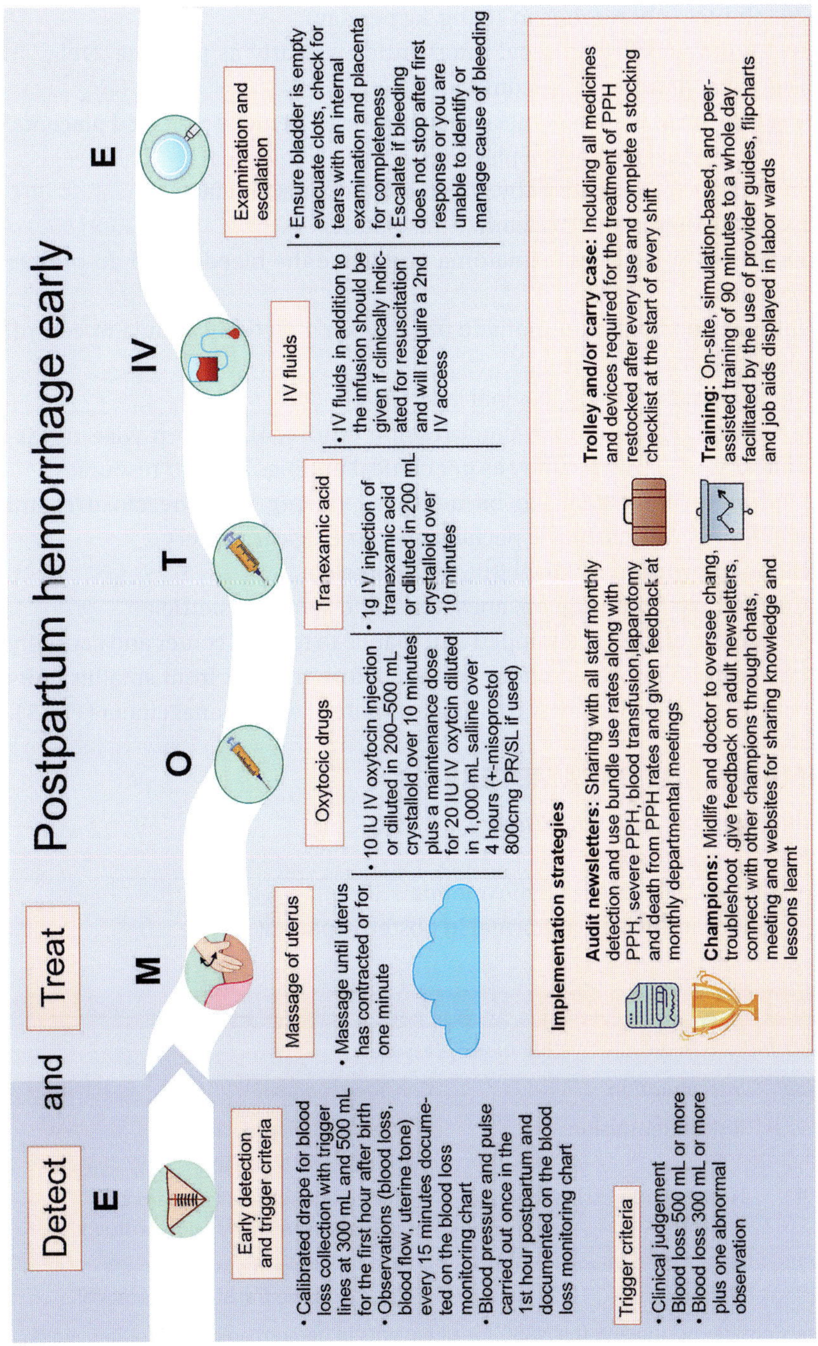

Fig. 3: Detect and treat PPH early.

- Start uterotonics if it atonic PPH and Tranexamic acid 1 gram IV slowly given within 3 hours of PPH is effective. It can be repeated after 30 minutes (not more than 10 mg/kg per day)
- In traumatic PPH, surgical intervention as early as possible. Delay in action will have poor outcome
- In PPH due to placental bits, evacuate uterus ,remove clots and placental bits or manual removal of placenta.
- In PPH due to coagulopathy, blood components and factor 7
- Evacuate uterus and catheterize the bladder
- Drain the episiotomy hematoma and ligate the bleeder and do presser packing
- Intrauterine ballon tamponade or Panicker's suction cannula to control atonic PPH
- Stitch cervical tear and vaginal laceration
- Other surgical options—compression suture, IIAL, step wise devascularization. Hysterectomy as per clinical findings and our resources
- Complete hemostasis to be achieved during uteri ne closure and abdominal wall closure especially inferior epigastric artery
- Blood transfusion protocol RBC:FPP:Platelets
- Call for help from surgeon, anesthetist and senior obstetrician
- Early referral in well-equipped ambulance to tertiary center and causality officer to be informed about patient before transfer from smaller units with less facility. Do not waste single minute of early management **(Fig. 3)**.

IMPORTANT PARAMETERS

- *Shock index = HR/SBP **(Table 1)**:*
  - Normal 0.5–0.7
  - Potential marker of hypovolemia
  - Shock index >0.9 abnormal in obstetric patient

TABLE 1: Clinical estimation using the shock index (SI).

Shock index = Heart rate/Systolic blood pressure		
Value	***Interpretation***	***Consider/suggest***
≥0.9	Risk of transfusion	• Aggressive approach • Transfer hemotransfusion
≥1.4	Need for aggressive therapy urgently	• Immediate aggressive approach • Open massive transfusion protocol
≥1.7	High risk of adverse maternal outcome	• Immediate aggressive approach • Open massive transfusion protocol

Note: Consider positioning the NASG for all patients in hemorrhagic shock or impending shock.
Source: OPAS. 208.

- *Modified shock index = HR/MAP:*
    - >1.3 is significant
    - Strong predictor of mortality in emergency
    - Shock index -no significant correlation with mortality

Rule of 30 to act fast:
- 30% loss of blood volume
- Systolic BP fall by 30 mm of Hg
- Heart rate rise by 30 beats/minute
- Resp rate by 30 breath/minute
- Urine output <30 mL/hour
- Hematocrit fall by 30%

SUGGESTED READING

1. Pacagnella RC, Borovac-Pinheiro A, Carla Silveira C, Morais SS, Argenton JLP, Souza JP, et al. The golden hour for postpartum hemorrhage: Results from a prospective cohort study. Int J Gyne and Obs. 2022;156(3):450-58.
2. National Institutes of Health (NIH) | (.gov) https://pubmed.ncbi.nlm.nih.gov › by RC Pacagnella. 2022.
3. Defines the golden hour in PPH. [online] Available from https://pmc.ncbi.nlm.nih.gov/articles/PMC10416182/National Institutes of Health (NIH) [Last acceessed January 2026].
4. The Global Library of Women's Medicine - Details the timeline and 4 Ts. [online] Available from https://www.glowm.com/article/heading/vol-13--obstetric-emergencies--nonconservative-and-conservative-surgical-management-of-pph/id/413063 [Last acceessed January 2026].
5. Discusses a multidisciplinary approach and "quantum acting". [online] Available from https://pmc.ncbi.nlm.nih.gov/articles/PMC11140635/National Institutes of Health (NIH) | (.gov) [Last acceessed January 2026].
6. Wiley - Study on vital signs during the golden hour. [online] Available from https://obgyn.onlinelibrary.wiley.com/doi/abs/10.1002/ijgo.13823 [Last acceessed January 2026].

15 CHAPTER

Placenta Accreta

Padma Shukla, Priyanshi Nigam

INTRODUCTION

Normally, the placenta anchors to decidualized endometrium whereas in placenta accreta, placental trophoblasts invade the myometrium abnormally due to defective decidualization. Placenta accreta, increta, and percreta are the spectrum of disorders that are classified as per the extent of myometrial invasion. It is associated with higher rates of maternal morbidity and mortality. Therefore, these patients should be taken care by multidisciplinary team. The International Federation of Gynecology and Obstetrics (FIGO) proposed a recent nomenclature of PAS that replaced the old terminology (placenta accreta, increta, and percreta) **(Fig. 1)**.

ETIOLOGY

Previous cesarean section is a major predisposing factor for the development of PAS disorders. Approximately 80% of placenta accreta cases are

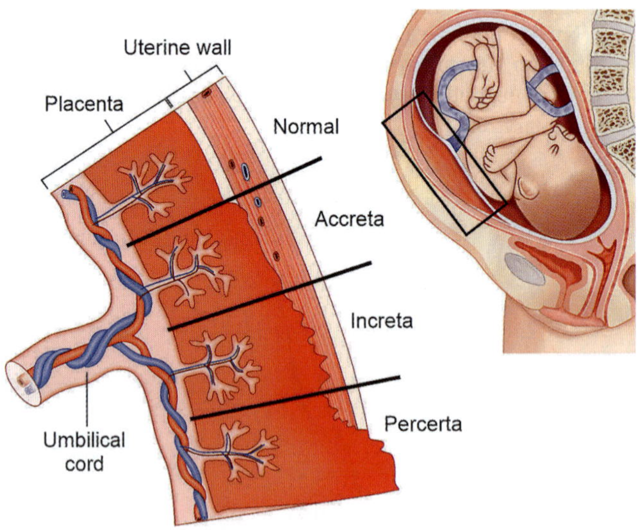

Fig. 1: Placenta accreta.

associated with placenta previa. Other risk factors associated with placenta accreta, include advanced maternal age, multiparity, uterine surgery, such as uterine curettage, myomectomy, prior endometrial ablation, hysteroscopic surgery, uterine embolization, pelvic irradiation and manual removal of placenta.

EPIDEMIOLOGY/INCIDENCE

The incidence of placenta accreta has dramatically increased from 1 in 533 pregnancies in the year 2000 to 1 in 272 in 2016 recent studies done in United states. The rise in cesarean section rates is a key contributor to the increasing occurrence of PAS, though cases have also been reported in women without prior uterine surgery or pregnancies.

PATHOPHYSIOLOGY

Recent evidence suggests that in some patients with prior uterine surgeries, abnormal decidualization in the area of uterine scar occurs due to absence of the spongiosus layer of the decidua. Furthermore, the main cause is not trophoblastic defect but abnormal endo-myometrial interface at site of implantation. The observed cellular alterations in the trophoblast are believed to result from the abnormal myometrial environment, rather than being due to an intrinsic defect in trophoblastic biology. Recent understanding suggests that PAS is not a truly invasive condition, as direct infiltration of surrounding organs by trophoblastic tissue has not been histologically confirmed. PAS is associated with formation of new blood vessels, which are delicate and prone to injury, lying deep in the pelvis leading to difficulty with surgical access and capable of large volume loss over a short time period. Also replacement of myometrium by scar tissue interferes in achieving hemostasis from placental bed. Hemorrhage and organ damage in attempt to stop bleeding is the main cause of morbidity.

CLINICAL FEATURES AND DIAGNOSIS

Usually this condition is asymptomatic but undiagnosed cases may present with hemorrhagic shock. Warning hemorrhage may be seen in some cases. Some women may present with heavy bleeding and passage of clots. Diagnosis is based on imaging that is 2D ultrasound and color Doppler. Accurate distinction between cases of placenta previa and placenta accreta with previa antenatally is crucial for pre-operative planning and counselling.

A systematic review suggests PAS remains undiagnosed in more than 50% cases. Ultrasonographic diagnostic features includes loss of retroplacental hypoechoic zone, myometrial thinning, increased vascularity, placental extension into serosa or bladder including bulge or focal exophytic mass.

Lacunae with turbulent blood flow may be seen in Color Doppler. A meta-analysis of ultrasound demonstrated a 90.8% sensitivity and 96.9% specificity. Important key diagnostic indicators include the presence of placental lacunae and loss of the hypoechoic retroplacental space. Diagnostic accuracy also depends significantly on the expertise of the sonologist.

Magnetic resonance imaging (MRI) has been widely employed, but as an adjunct to ultrasound. A systematic review demonstrates 94.4% sensitivity and 84.0% specificity rates for diagnosis with MRI. In India, facilities performing MRI for obstetric indications must be registered under the PCPNDT Act.

Some studies suggested that AFP can be used as potential predictor for placenta accreta, with a threshold value of ≥2.5 MoM demonstrating a sensitivity of 86.8% and a specificity of 72.1%.

FIGO CLASSIFICATION OF PAS (FIG. 2)

- *Grade 1 (accreta):* Focal adherence without significant invasion into myometrium.
- *Grade 2 (increta):* Invasion into myometrium but not reaching the serosa.
- *Grade 3a (percreta):* Invasion through myometrium and up to serosa, but not through it.
- *Grade 3b:* Invasion into adjacent bladder.
- *Grade 3c:* Invasion into other pelvic organs (e.g., bowel and parametrium)

Another classification is focal partial and complete according to the area of involvement of myometrium.

MANAGEMENT

Antenatal diagnosis of placenta accreta spectrum is associated with reduced hemorrhage and better maternal and fetal prognosis. Irrespective of prenatal diagnosis hysterectomy rates were >50%. The American College of Obstetricians and Gynecologists (ACOG) has recommended delivery between 34 0/7 and 35 6/7 weeks of gestation via planned cesarean hysterectomy after steroid coverage. Patients diagnosed with PAS should be referred to a Placenta Accreta Center of Excellence (PACE) or a Level 3 or 4 facility for delivery, where multidisciplinary teams are available to optimize outcomes. These teams should include perinatologists, pelvic surgeons, intensivists, general surgeons, urologists, and neonatologists. Detailed consent including ICU stay, injury to adjacent organs, risk of massive hemorrhage, multiple transfusions, ventilatory support, emergency hysterectomy is mandatory.

ACOG RECOMMENDATION 2018 (TABLE 1)

TABLE 1: Recommendations regarding management of placenta accreta spectrum.

Recommendation	*Grade of recommendation*
Diagnosis of placenta accreta spectrum	
Although ultrasound evaluation is important. The absence of ultrasound findings does not preclude a diagnosis of PAS; thus, clinical risk factors remain equally important as predictors of PAS by ultrasound findings	IA Strong recommendation, high-quality evidence
It is unclear whether MRI improves diagnosis of PAS beyond that achieved with ultrasonography alone. Accordingly, MRI is not the preferred recommended modality for the initial evaluation of possible PAS	1B Strong recommendation, moderate-quality evidence
Women with suspected PAS diagnosed in the antenatal period based on imaging or by clinical acumen should be delivered at a level III or IV center with considerable experience whenever possible to improve outcomes	1B Strong recommendation, moderate-quality evidence
Management	
Optimal management involves a standardized approach with a comprehensive multidisciplinary care team accustomed to management of PAS	1B Strong recommendation, moderate-quality evidence
Delivery at 34 0/7–35 6/7 weeks of gestation is suggested as the preferred gestational age for scheduled cesarean delivery or hysterectomy absent extenuating circumstances in a stable patient. Earlier delivery may be required in cases of persistent bleeding preeclampsia, labor, rupture of membranes, fetal compromise, or developing maternal comorbidities	IA Strong recommendation, high-quality evidence
In the setting of hemorrhage, data from other surgical disciplines support the use of a range of 1:1:1 to 1:2:4 strategy of packed red blood cells: fresh frozen plasma: platelets	IA Strong recommendation, high-quality evidence
Conservative management or expectant management should be considered only for carefully selected cases of PAS after detailed counseling about the risks. uncertain benefits. and efficacy and should be considered investigational	2C Weak recommendation, low-quality evidence

Strategies to reduce hemorrhage-related morbidity and mortality include the early administration of intravenous tranexamic acid, preoperative autologous blood donation and implementation of massive transfusion protocols using a 1:1:1 ratio of packed red blood cells, fresh frozen plasma, and platelets.

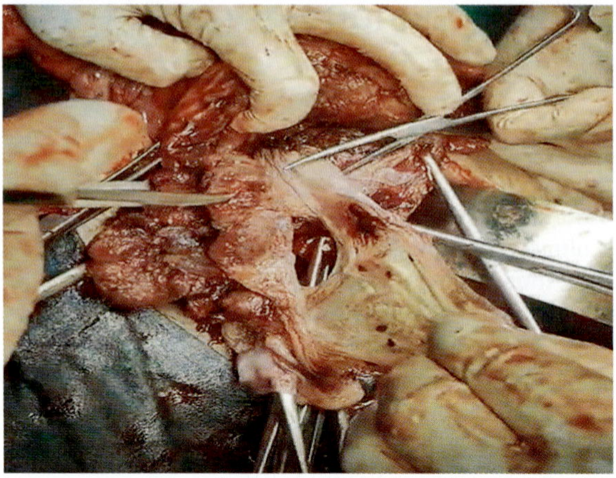

Fig. 2: Placenta accreta spectrum.

Preoperative Evaluation and Preparation

All blood investigation, preop checkup, anesthetic detailed evaluation and a detailed ultrasonography for localization of placenta, its boundaries and extension to adjacent tissue should be noted. MRI and cystoscopy should be performed, if required.

CONSERVATIVE MANAGEMENT

It is associated with reduced surgical morbidity and may offer an effective alternative to cesarean hysterectomy. Conservative management requires careful patient selection and close monitoring. Conservative management is done in relatively hemodynamically stable cases of partial or focal accreta, who wants to preserve fertility and is available for close follow-up.

Methods

Leaving Placenta In Situ

This method involves delivering the fetus while intentionally retaining the placenta in situ, with partial or complete adherence to the myometrium, thereby preventing the need for hysterectomy in 78 to 80% of cases. The progressive decrease in blood supply to the uterus after delivery results in placental necrosis and detachment, followed by placental resorption and expulsion. The tissue may take 6 months to get resorbed. Serial monitoring with beta-hCG and USG is required. Administration of methotrexate systemically led to decreased placental mass and reduced uteroplacental blood flow. However, this method is associated with a morbidity rate of 56–87.5%, and complications such as postpartum hemorrhage, infection, sepsis, disseminated intravascular coagulation, delayed hysterectomy.

Triple-P Procedure

The triple P procedure is comprised of three essential steps: Perioperative placental ultrasound localization, pelvic devascularization involving pre-operative placement of intra-arterial balloon catheters (anterior division of the internal iliac arteries) and no attempt to remove the entire placenta with large myometrial excision and uterine repair. This procedure is contra-indicated in cases of percreta with lateral extension.

Modified triple P procedure, include temporary clamping of the internal iliac arteries, ligation of internal iliac arteries, and the application of a tourniquet around the lower uterine segment to reduce the vascularity prior to myometrial excision.

Compression Sutures

Compression sutures like cervico-isthmic sutures, P-sutures, and easy Gideon sutures are also very helpful in preventing hemorrhage and thus reducing morbidity and mortality.

P-suture is an innovative suture applied through the lateral myometrial wall of the uterus **(Fig. 3)**. Suture is applied 1 cm medial to the lateral border of uterus, taking stitch anterior to posterior from one side and bringing same stitch posterior to anterior from another side and ligating anteriorly. This results in approximation of anterior and posterior uterine wall and thereby effective hemostasis in placenta accreta. The principle of this suture is compression of arcuate and spiral arterioles at the site of hemorrhage. Wide application of sutures can be done from lower segment to fundus, depending on the location and extent of bleeding. In cases where P-sutures become loose following placental removal, they may be re-tied and secured again to ensure adequate hemostasis.

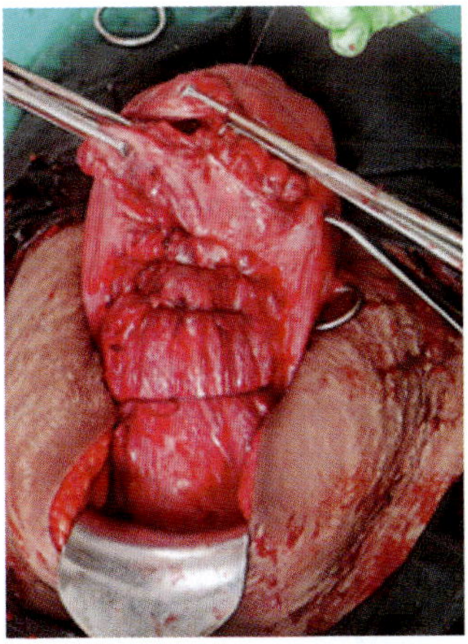

Fig. 3: P-sutures in case of PAS.

Easy Gideon sutures were placed using Vicryl 1-0, passed through the avascular areas of the broad ligament, medial to the round ligaments—anterior to posterior on one side and posterior to anterior on the other—and tied anteriorly, thereby approximating the uterine walls and compressing the uterine arteries to control bleeding.

Cervico-isthmic sutures—the uterus was exteriorized, after reflecting bladder downwards, a No. 2 chromic catgut suture on a straight needle was placed approximately 3 cm below the uterine incision and 2 cm medial to the lateral edge of the lower segment. The suture was passed from the anterior to the posterior uterine wall and returned 1 cm medial to the entry point, then tied anteriorly. A closed artery forceps was inserted through the uterine incision into the cervical canal to maintain patency. The procedure was repeated symmetrically on the contralateral side.

Interval Hysterectomy

It is a good alternative preventing complications occurring in immediate hysterectomy and prolonged retained placenta. A better plane of dissection can be seen, thus reducing risk of bladder injuries. Risk of DIC, infection and hemorrhage.

Surgical Management

Complete cesarean hysterectomy is the gold standard delivery method for women with PAS.

Steps

- Abdomen opened by midline vertical incision
- Hysterotomy done 2 cm above from the placental edge, avoiding incising the placenta thus preventing massive hemorrhage.
- Uterotonics should be administered after delivery of fetus
- Hysterotomy should be closed, leaving placenta in situ and then proceeding for hysterectomy
- A newer concept of retrograde hysterectomy has been put forward to prevent bladder injury. After cutting and ligating the round ligaments, one assistant will direct his fingers through vagina to identify the posterior vaginal fornix, posterior vagina is then incised and uterosacral ligaments are divided after which lateral fornices are incised to cut the cardinal ligaments. After which the bladder is lifted from below upwards and anterior vaginal opened and ligation of vesicouterine vessels done following removal of uterus and cervix and vault closure done after achieving hemostasis. Inspection of the pelvic area should be done for hemostasis before closing the abdomen.

PROGNOSIS

The prognosis is better for patients who have placenta accreta without placenta previa. Placenta accreta with previa has a higher risk of hemorrhage and is more likely to undergo a hysterectomy, both of which contribute to morbidity. Patients who have Grade 3 invasion have more complications as compared to grade 1 and 2.

COMPLICATIONS

In the majority of placenta accreta cases intrapartum hemorrhage is the most common complication. One study suggests, 80% patients necessitated transfusions and 28% cases went into DIC. Hemorrhage is best reduced if the placenta is left in situ after fetal delivery, as noted previously; however, it is often not avoidable.

The major complications include injury to adjacent organs like bladder, ureter and bowel. Inadvertent or intentional cystotomy can occur during the procedure especially in previous cesarean sections. Most commonly, it is associated with anterior placenta previa, which may require cystostomy for placental tissue separation. Ureteral injury usually occurs due to the technical difficulty of a cesarean hysterectomy. Adequate counselling of the patient for these complications is mandatory. Maternal hemorrhage often leads to preterm delivery and worsens neonatal outcomes.

POINTS TO REMEMBER

1. Placenta accreta spectrum (PAS) arises from abnormal placental adherence to the myometrium, primarily due to defective decidualization with absence of the decidua basalis and its spongiosus layer.
2. Risk factors include prior cesarean section, placenta previa, multiparity, prior uterine surgery, curettage, etc.
3. Most cases are asymptomatic, diagnosis is mainly dependent on imaging like 2D-ultrasound and color Doppler.
4. FIGO has classified PAS into Grade 1, 2, 3a, 3b, 3c depending upon grade of invasion.
5. Delivery should be planned between 34+0/7 to 35+6/7 weeks in PACE centers or tertiary care centers with a multidisciplinary team after steroid coverage.
6. Conservative management includes leaving placenta in situ, triple P procedure, interval hysterectomy and compression sutures like P-sutures, easy Gideon sutures, cervico-isthmic sutures.
7. In spite of antenatal diagnosis, hysterectomy is performed in more than 50% of cases.
8. Complications are massive hemorrhage (~80% need transfusion), DIC (~28%), injury to bladder/ureter/bowel, infection, preterm delivery.
9. Prognosis better in accreta without previa, worse with higher grades of invasion.

SUGGESTED READING

1. Abbas RA, Nassar AH. Placenta Accreta Spectrum: Conservative Management and Its Impact on Future Fertility. Matern Fetal Med. 2021;3(4):263-7.

2. Abouda HS, Aloui H, Azouz E, Marzouk SB, Frikha H, Hammami R, et al. New surgical technique for managing placenta accreta spectrum and pilot study of the "CMNT PAS" study. AJOG Glob Rep. 2025;5(1):100430.
3. Adler E, Madankumar R, Rosner M, Reznik SE. Increased placental trophoblast inclusions in placenta accreta. Placenta. 2014;35(12):1075-8.
4. Adu-Bredu TK, Rijken MJ, Nieto-Calvache AJ, Stefanovic V, Aryananda RA, Fox KA, et al. A simple guide to ultrasound screening for placenta accreta spectrum for improving detection and optimizing management in resource limited settings. Int J Gynecol Obstet. 2023;160:732-41.
5. American College of Obstetricians and Gynecologists; Society for Maternal-Fetal Medicine. Obstetric Care Consensus No. 7: Placenta Accreta Spectrum. Obstet Gynecol. 2018;132(6):e259-75.
6. Bhanumathy P, Balachandran DM, Cleetus N, Hassan J, Pappachan S, G KL. Caesarean Hysterectomy for Placenta Accreta Spectrum in a Single Centre: A Series of 19 Cases. Eur Med J. 2024.
7. Bowman ZS, Eller AG, Kennedy AM, Richards DS, Winter TC, Woodward PJ, et al. Accuracy of ultrasound for the prediction of placenta accreta. Am J Obstet Gynecol. 2014;211(2):177.e1-7.
8. Dedes I, Ziogas V. Circular isthmic-cervical sutures can be an alternative method to control peripartum haemorrhage during caesarean section for placenta praevia accreta. Arch Gynecol Obstet. 2008;278(6):555-7.
9. D'Antonio F, Iacovella C, Palacios-Jaraquemada J, Bruno CH, Manzoli L, Bhide A. Prenatal identification of invasive placentation using magnetic resonance imaging: systematic review and meta-analysis. Ultrasound Obstet Gynecol. 2014;44(1):8-16.
10. Eller AG, Porter TF, Soisson P, Silver RM. Optimal management strategies for placenta accreta. BJOG. 2009;116(5):648-54.
11. Grace Tan SE, Jobling TW, Wallace EM, McNeilage LJ, Manolitsas T, Hodges RJ. Surgical management of placenta accreta: a 10-year experience. Acta Obstet Gynecol Scand. 2013;92(4):445-50.
12. Hecht JL, Baergen R, Ernst LM, Katzman PJ, Jacques SM, Jauniaux E, et al. Classification and reporting guidelines for the pathology diagnosis of placenta accreta spectrum (PAS) disorders: recommendations from an expert panel. Mod Pathol. 2020;33(12):2382-96.
13. Japaraj RP, Mimin TS, Mukudan K. Antenatal diagnosis of placenta previa accreta in patients with previous cesarean scar. J Obstet Gynaecol Res. 2007; 33(4):431-7.
14. Khong TY. The pathology of placenta accreta, a worldwide epidemic. J Clin Pathol. 2008;61(12):1243-6.
15. Lee PS, Kempner S, Miller M, Dominguez J, Grotegut C, Ehrisman J, et al. Multidisciplinary approach to manage antenatally suspected placenta percreta: updated algorithm and patient outcomes. Gynecol Oncol Res Pract. 2017;4:11.
16. Mappa I, Espuelas Malon S, D'Antonio F, Chandraharan E. Effectiveness of the Triple P Procedure and its modifications on reducing the blood loss and peripartum hysterectomy rates in women with Placenta Accreta Spectrum (PAS): a review of published literature. J Matern Fetal Neonatal Med. 2025; 38(1):2452920.

17. Mogos MF, Salemi JL, Ashley M, Whiteman VE, Salihu HM. Recent trends in placenta accreta in the United States and its impact on maternal-fetal morbidity and healthcare-associated costs, 1998-2011. J Matern Fetal Neonatal Med. 2016;29(7):1077-82.
18. Mulla BM, Weatherford R, Redhunt AM, Modest AM, Hacker MR, Hecht JL, et al. Hemorrhagic morbidity in placenta accreta spectrum with and without placenta previa. Arch Gynecol Obstet. 2019;300(6):1601-6.
19. Pekar Zlotin M, Sharabi-Nov A, Meiri H, Revivo PE, Melcer Y, Maymon R, et al. Clinical-sonographic scores for the screening of placenta accreta spectrum: a systematic review and meta-analysis. Am J Obstet Gynecol MFM. 2024;6(8):101369.
20. Riteau AS, Tassin M, Chambon G, Le Vaillant C, de Laveaucoupet J, Quéré MP, et al. Accuracy of ultrasonography and magnetic resonance imaging in the diagnosis of placenta accreta. PLoS One. 2014;9(4):e94866.
21. Sentilhes L, Kayem G, Chandraharan E, Palacios-Jaraquemada J, Jauniaux E. FIGO consensus guidelines on placenta accreta spectrum disorders: conservative management. Int J Gynecol Obstet. 2018;140(3):291-8.
22. Shah SR, Chudasama TJ, Patel BS, Vyas RC, Parikh PM, Dodiya HN, et al. Placenta Accreta Spectrum (PAS) disorders: A 10-year study at tertiary care center, Ahmedabad, Western India. Int J Clin Obstet Gynaecol. 2020;4(4): 161-6.
23. Sharma K. Easy Gideon Suture vs Cervico-Isthmic Suture with Bilateral Uterine Artery Compression Suture in Management of PPH in a Tertiary Care Hospital of Bihar. Int J Res Eng Sci. 2021;9(10):1-5.
24. Silver RM, Landon MB, Rouse DJ, Leveno KJ, Spong CY, Thom EA, et al.; National Institute of Child Health and Human Development Maternal-Fetal Medicine Units Network. Maternal morbidity associated with multiple repeat cesarean deliveries. Obstet Gynecol. 2006;107(6):1226-32.
25. Singh Y, Raghav V, Kapur A. Medical Management of Placenta Accreta with Methotrexate: Review of Two Cases. J South Asian Feder Obst Gynae. 2015; 7(2):86-8.
26. Su HW, Yi YC, Tseng JJ, Chen WC, Chen YF, Kung HF, et al. Maternal outcome after conservative management of abnormally invasive placenta. Taiwan J Obstet Gynecol. 2017;56(3):353-7.
27. Takeda S, Takeda J, Murayama Y. Placenta Previa Accreta Spectrum: Cesarean Hysterectomy. Surg J (N Y). 2021;7(Suppl 1):S28-S37.
28. WOMAN Trial Collaborators. Effect of early tranexamic acid administration on mortality, hysterectomy, and other morbidities in women with post-partum haemorrhage (WOMAN): an international, randomised, double-blind, placebo-controlled trial. Lancet. 2017;389(10084):2105-16.
29. Zelop C, Nadel A, Frigoletto FD Jr, Pauker S, MacMillan M, Benacerraf BR. Placenta accreta/percreta/increta: a cause of elevated maternal serum alpha-fetoprotein. Obstet Gynecol. 1992;80(4):693-4.

16 CHAPTER

Active Management of Third Stage of Labor

Ishika Nain

INTRODUCTION

The third stage of labor is the duration between the delivery of the baby and the expulsion of the placenta. The duration of the third stage of labor is about 6 to 30 minutes.

Management goals of third stage includes delivering an intact placenta and avoiding uterine inversion or postpartum hemorrhage. Currently two methods are in practice:

1. Expectant management
2. Active management of third stage of labor (AMTSL)

EXPECTANT MANAGEMENT

In this, the placental separation and its descent into the vagina are allowed to occur spontaneously or aided by nipple stimulation or gravity (World Health Organization 2012). Minimal assistance may be given for placental expulsion if needed. Immediately after newborn birth, uterine fundal size and consistency are examined. If the uterus remains firm and bleeding is minimal, watchful waiting until the placenta separates is the usual practice. Neither massage nor downward fundal pressure is employed, but the fundus is frequently palpated to ensure that it does not become atonic and filled with blood from placental separation. To prevent uterine inversion, umbilical cord traction must not be used to pull the placenta from the uterus.

Signs of separation include:

1. Sudden gush of blood into the vagina,
2. A globular and firmer fundus,
3. Outward movement of the umbilical cord as the placenta descends into the vagina, and elevation of the uterus into the abdomen.

These signs appear within minutes after newborn delivery, and the median time ranges from 4 to 12 minutes. Once the placenta has detached from the uterine wall, the mother can bear down, and intra-abdominal pressure often expels the placenta into the vagina. After ensuring that the uterus is contracted firmly, the umbilical cord is kept slightly taut but is not pulled. Pressure is exerted by a hand wrapped around the fundus to propel the detached placenta into the vagina. Concurrently, the heel of the same hand exerts pressure between the symphysis pubis and the uterine fundus and directs it toward the sacrum. This aims to prevent inversion. Once the placenta passes through the introitus, pressure on the uterus is relieved. The placenta is then gently lifted away. Care is taken to prevent placental membranes from being torn off and left behind. If the membranes begin to tear, they are grasped with a clamp and removed by gentle teasing.

ACTIVE MANAGEMENT OF THIRD STAGE OF LABOR

Active management of third stage of labor is a prophylactic, deliberate, effective intervention to ensure smooth expulsion of the placenta and prevention of postpartum hemorrhage. It has been recommended by World Health Organization since 2007 for prevention of postpartum hemorrhage. It has three components:

1. Administration of a uterotonic, preferably oxytocin, immediately after birth of the baby
2. Controlled cord traction (CCT) to deliver the placenta; and
3. Massage of the uterine fundus after the placenta is delivered

   The goal of this triad is to limit postpartum hemorrhage.

ADMINISTRATION OF UTEROTONIC DRUGS

A single agent is given either before or after placental expulsion, and timing does not affect rates of postpartum hemorrhage, placental retention, or third-stage labor length.

In 2012, the results of a large WHO-directed, multicentered clinical trial were published and showed that the most important AMTSL component was the administration of a uterotonic.

Choices for hemorrhage prophylaxis include oxytocin, misoprostol, and the ergots, namely ergonovine and methylergonovine. In addition, a combination agent of oxytocin plus ergonovine is also used. Also in India, carbetocin, a long-acting oxytocin analog, is available and effective for hemorrhage prevention. Of agents, the WHO (2018) recommends oxytocin for first-line use. High-dose synthetic oxytocin is identical to that produced by the posterior pituitary.

The dosage of various uterotonic as per international guidelines are listed in the **Table 1** below.

The dosage of uterotonics as per FOGSI GCPR 2014 are as follows **(Table 2)**.

Controlled Cord Traction

Clamp the cord close to the perineum. Place the other hand just above the woman's pubic bone and stabilize the uterus. Hold the cord and await

TABLE 1: The dosage of various uterotonic as per international guidelines.

	ACOG	*RANZCOG*	*RCOG*	*SCOG*
Oxytocin	10–40 IU IV or 10 IU IM	Not specific	5 IU IV (repeatable)	10 IU IM or 5 IU IV or 40 IU IV 125 mL/h in 500 mL
Ergots	Methylergonovine 0.2 mg IM per 24 h period	Not specific	Ergometrine 0.5 mg IV or IM	Ergonovine 0.25 mg IV or IM every 2 h
Misoprostol	800–1,000 µg rectal	1,000 µg rectal	1,000 µg rectal	400–1,000 µg oral or rectal
Tranexamic acid	–	–	Not suggested	Not suggested

(ACOG: American Congress of Obstetrics and Gynecology; RANZCOG: Royal Australian and New Zealand Congress of Obstetrics and Gynecology; RCOG: Royal Congress of Obstetrics and Gynecology; SCOG: Canadian Society Obstetrics and Gynecology; IV: intravenous; IM: intramuscular)

TABLE 2: The dosage of uterotonics as per FOGSI GCPR 2014.

Drug	*Dosage route of administration*	*Action*	*Side effects*	*Caution*
Oxytocin	• 10 U IM • 5 U IV diluted to 5 mL over 1–2 mins slow • 20 U in 500 mL NS/RL infusion @ 150 mL/hour	• Onset 2–3 mins • *Lasts up to:* 15–20 mins	None or minimal	Direct IV oxytocin contra indicated in cases of cardio-vascular failure and heart diseases
Misoprostol	600 mcg oral/SL/PR	• Onset 3–5 mins • Peak 20–30 mins • *Last up to:* 75 mins	Shivering, slight rise in temperature	No contra-indications
Ergometrine	0.2 mg IM	• *Onset:* 1–2 mins • Lasts 2–4 hours	May increase risk of retained placenta, nausea vomiting, head-ache, hypertension	Avoid in hypertension, heart disease, Rh negative mothers
Carboprost	250 mcg IM	• *Onset:* 1–2 mins • Lasts 15–20 mins	Vomiting, diarrhea, bronchospasm	Avoid bronchial asthma

a strong uterine contraction (2–3 minutes). Pull the cord downwards with continuous counter pressure on the uterus directed upwards and deliver the placenta. If the placenta does not descend during 30–40 seconds of controlled cord traction do not continue to pull on the cord. Wait until the uterus is well contracted again and repeat procedure.

'Never apply cord traction (pull down) without applying counter pressure (push up)'. As the placenta delivers hold the placenta in two hands and gently turn it until membranes are twisted. Slowly pull to complete the delivery. Examine the maternal and the fetal surface of the placenta and the membranes. If a portion of the maternal surface is missing or there are torn membranes with vessels, suspect retained placenta fragments and take appropriate action.

The WHO trial conducted in 2012 also demonstrated that the addition of CCT did almost nothing to reduce hemorrhage. The women who received CCT bled 10 mL less (on average) than women who delivered their placenta by their own effort. There was a real difference, however, in terms of the length of the third stage: third stage was an average of six minutes longer among those women who did not receive CCT.

Massage of Uterine Fundus

Uterine fundus should me massaged immediately after delivery of placenta. Palpate for a contracted uterus every 15 minutes for one hour. Repeat uterine massage as needed. Ensure that the uterus does not become relaxed (soft) after you stop uterine massage.

A refocused approach to prevention of PPH Using AMTSL as proposed by WHO in 2012

- *Uterotonic:* Ensure that every woman is offered a uterotonic immediately after the delivery of the baby. Oxytocin is the preferred drug to prevent PPH.
- *Delayed cord clamping:* Delay clamping the cord for at least 1–3 minutes to reduce rates of infant anemia.
- *CCT:* Perform CCT, if required. In settings where skilled birth attendants are unavailable, CCT is not recommended. CCT is the recommended method for removal of the placenta in caesarean section.
- *Postpartum vigilance:* Immediately assess uterine tone to ensure a contracted uterus; continue to check every 15 minutes for 2 hours. If there is uterine atony, perform fundal massage and monitor more frequently.
- *Oxytocin quality and supply:* Ensure a continuous supply of high-quality oxytocin. Maintain the cool chain for oxytocin, and remember that potency is reduced if oxytocin is exposed to heat for long periods.

SUGGESTED READING

1. Cunningham FG, Leveno KJ, Dashe JS, Hoffman BL, Spong CY, Casey BM. Williams Obstetrics 26th edition. Philadelphia: McGraw Hill; 2022.
2. FOGSI. (2014). Prevention of Post Partum Hemorrhage (PPH) Consensus Statement for Prevention of PPH Reviewed at the Consensus group meeting at Amby Valley. [online] Available from https://www.fogsi.org/wp-content/uploads/2015/11/pph.pdf [Last accessed December, 2025].
3. Güngördük K, Olgaç Y, Gülseren V, Kocaer M. Active management of the third stage of labor: A brief overview of key issues. Turk J Obstet Gynecol. 2018;15(3):188-92.
4. WHO. (2012). WHO recommendations for active management of third stage of labour. [online] Available from https://iris.who.int/server/api/core/bitstreams/c71a1c3a-5df3-43f3-8993-b5300116578e/content [Last accessed December, 2025].

17 CHAPTER

Role of Uterine Massage and Aortic Compression in Management of Postpartum Hemorrhage

Aditi Rathore

INTRODUCTION

Maternal hemorrhage remains the leading cause of maternal mortality worldwide. ACOG reVITALize program defines cumulative blood loss greater than or equal to 1,000 mL or blood loss accompanied by signs or symptoms of hypovolemia within 24 hours after the birth process (includes intrapartum blood loss) regardless of route of delivery.

PPH occurs in approximately 1 to 3% of all deliveries and is the leading cause of obstetric morbidity and mortality worldwide. In India, PPH, which is exacerbated by widespread anemia among pregnant women, accounts for 38 percent of maternal deaths.

Primary PPH occurs within 24 hours postpartum, while secondary PPH happens after 24 hours and up to 12 weeks later. The main causes are summarized by the 4 "T's" (tone, trauma, tissue, thrombin) and require prompt intervention. Uterine atony is the major cause of PPH and accounts for 70% of total cases.

Management involves an interprofessional approach, emphasizing accurate blood loss assessment, fluid replacement, and source control.

In the past 20 years, a set of cost-effective interventions, suitable for implementation at both health center and hospital level, have been developed. Some of these can also be used in the community or at home. We thus have another set of tools to control moderate and severe post-partum hemorrhaging (PPH). The use of these tools is also increasingly being combined in a standardized and simplified approach.

The World Health Organization (WHO) hosted an expert consultation on PPH bundles in December 2017, where a consensus was found that every port partum hemorrhage should be treated rapidly

The following set of actions were agreed at a World Health Organization expert consultation on PPH bundles in 2017.

BUNDLE 1

This is a standardized treatment approach for every case of PPH, comprising four actions, designed to be carried out at the same time:

- Uterotonics
- Uterine massage

- Tranexamic acid (TXA)
- IV fluids (crystalloids)

BUNDLE 2

This offers a further set of actions for teams working with a woman who, in spite of interventions, continues to bleed profusely ('refractory bleeding'):

- Bimanual uterine massage
- Aorta compression
- Non-pneumatic anti-shock garment (NASG)
- Uterine balloon tamponade (UBT)

MANAGEMENT

The main approach is patient resuscitation and identifying and treating the underlying cause.

Clinicians should be prepared to use a combination of pharmacological, mechanical and surgical methods to arrest PPH. These methods should be directed towards the causative factor.

When uterine atony is perceived to be a cause of the bleeding, then a sequence of mechanical and pharmacological measures should be instituted in turn until the bleeding stops.

Zero-hour Checklist

- Once a woman has been assessed to have PPH, call the Emergency Response Team (ERT) for help.
- Initial resuscitation with ABCDE (airway, breathing, circulation, disability, exposure) approach is to be done.
- IV access with two wide bore cannula #14/16
- Blood sample for investigations to be collected and adequate blood and blood products to be arranged.
- Catheterization is mandatory.
- The vitals—shock index must be recorded.
- Quick history and rapid initial assessment

Clinical and Pharmacological Management

- Ensure the cause by palpating the uterus for atony.
- In cases of uterine atony, the primary response is to do uterine massage, bimanual uterine compression, aortic compression, and administer uterotonics.
- *Tranexamic acid injection:* 1 g IV to be given immediately (within 3 hours of PPH) and repeat another 1 g IV after 30 minutes if PPH persists.
- If the uterus has contracted, inspect for genital tract trauma. If detected, appropriate intervention should be taken.

- Evaluate for blood coagulation abnormalities.
- If patient is still bleeding and goes in refractory PPH then, bimanual uterine compression, aortic compression, uterine balloon tamponade to be done and NASG to be placed.
- In cases of lower level health facilities, transfer and appropriate referral to be done.
- In level II and level III settings, if women is still bleeding, she can be taken for surgical compression sutures, uterine artery ligation (stepwise devascularization), uterine artery embolization, and hysterectomy.

Uterine massage and external aortic compression are simple, non-expensive techniques which can be applied in low-resourced settings to prevent or treat PPH.

Uterine Massage

Uterine massage is a recognized method to manage postpartum hemorrhage due to atonic uterus. Uterine massage after delivery of the placenta promotes contraction of the uterus.

Uterine Massage Technique

To perform uterine massage in the prehospital environment, one hand is placed just above the symphysis pubis to support the lower uterine segment while the other hand is placed on top of the fundus, firmly massaging it in a circular motion towards the supporting hand. This should be repeated every 10 minutes during transport if bleeding is continuing, or the uterus feels "spongey", "boggy" or soft rather than firm like a basketball. Clots may be expelled during contraction. The mother should also be encouraged to breastfeed the newborn as this will help to stimulate uterine contractions **(Fig. 1)**.

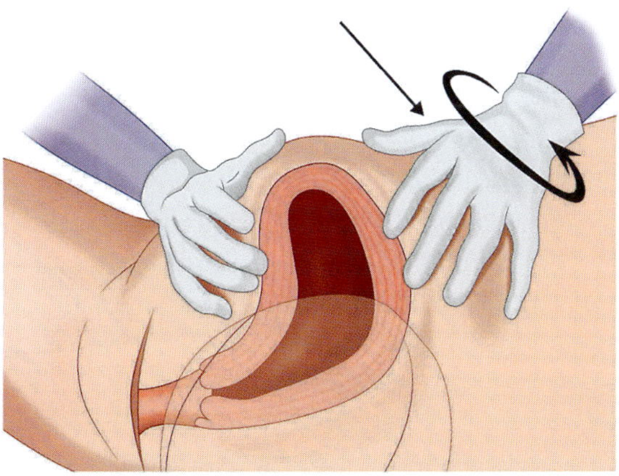

Fig. 1: Uterine massage technique.

Bimanual Uterine Compression

Two hands are used one in the anterior vaginal fornix and one behind the uterus, squeezing the uterus between the two hands. This is to be used if uterus fails to contract after 2 doses of uterotonics and uterine massage **(Fig. 2)**.

Uterine massage is a known recommended part of AMTSL and also a part of first response bundle for PPH.

As a general preventive approach, the existing GOI guideline strongly recommend the use of oxytocin for active management of the third stage of labor (along with other two steps: CCT and uterine massage), because it reduces PPH by more than 60%.

Guidelines for the prevention of postpartum hemorrhage, such as the joint statement of the International Confederation of Midwives and the International Federation of Gynecology and Obstetrics, recommend routine massage of the uterus after delivery of the placenta. Massage is thought to stimulate uterine contraction, possibly through stimulation of local prostaglandin release, and thus reduce hemorrhage. However, there has been very little empirical research to evaluate the effectiveness of this method.

However sustained uterine massage, started before delivery of the placenta, in reducing postpartum hemorrhage has not shown any advantage.

External Aortic Compression

External aortic compression is an emergency maneuver designed to reduce postpartum hemorrhage and allow time for resuscitation and to control the bleeding. It involves manually pressing down on the abdomen to stem the flow of blood through the aorta to the vagina. Compressing the aorta, by applying firm pressure with a closed fist just above the umbilicus, slows bleeding **(Fig. 3)**.

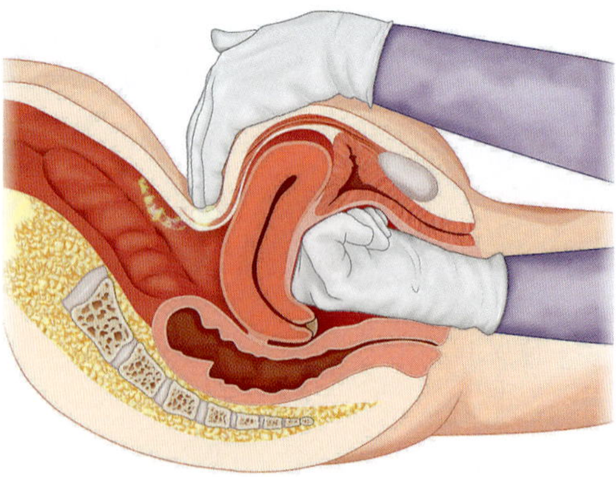

Fig. 2: Bimanual uterine compression.

It is recommended in cases of severe life-threatening postpartum hemorrhage-particularly when a patient is being stabilized or transported. It may be used as an adjunct to other measures, especially in locations or situations where there is no access to advanced medical assistance **(Fig. 4)**.

The theory is that abdominal compression will decrease blood flow in the distal aorta, helping to control bleeding in the pelvis and extremities. Enough pressure is applied and it is confirmed by the disappearance of femoral pulsation to be confirmed by an assistant. In one report, 80 to 140 lb of pressure applied to the epigastrium in 9 healthy male participants in a supine position on a rigid surface resulted in decreased blood flow in the common femoral artery as determined by pulsed-wave Doppler ultrasound. Abdominal pressure applied above the umbilicus also has been reported to

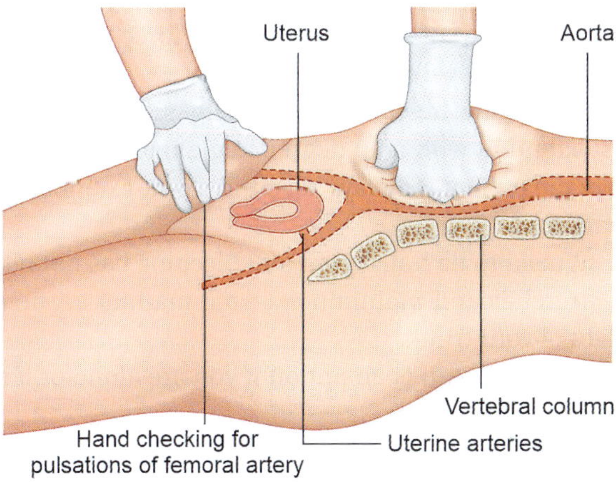

Fig. 3: External aortic compression.

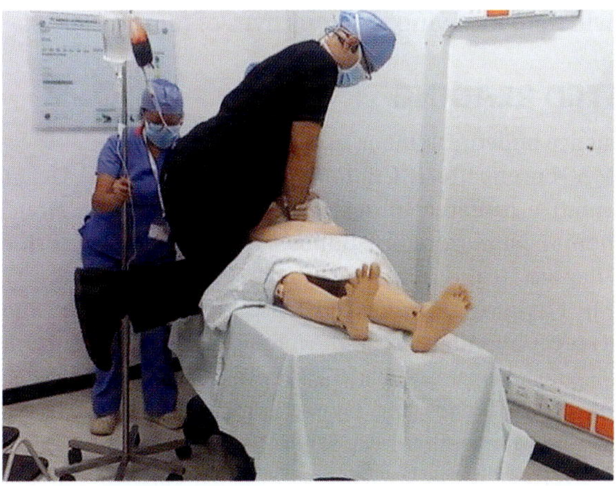

Fig. 4: Advanced medical assistance.

reduce blood pressure in the legs. Abdominal compression and tourniquets used on the extremities are not meant to be definitive treatments for traumatic hemorrhages but rather are used to stabilize severely injured patients during transport to emergency surgical care facilities.

Using manual compression, it is difficult for a clinician to exert the equivalent of 140 lb on the epigastrium for the extended period of time needed to transport an injured person to an emergency facility. Therefore, mechanical devices such as the abdominal aortic tourniquet (AAT) and the nonpneumatic antishock garment (NASG) have been developed to aid in providing continuous abdominal compression.

Ideally do not attempt to compress the aorta with the strength of your arm it will lead to tiredness and the compression will be ineffective leading to recurrent bleeding. Position yourself beside the patient and use a step stool if needed to achieve a height that allows you to compress effectively.

Administer the weight of your trunk not the force of your arms onto the patient abdomen at the level of the navel.

This maneuver may be painful so analgesia can be given. Ensure your elbow is extended with a 90 degree angle between your arm and the stretcher where the patient is always keep the elbow extended, back straight, and knees straight.

If the patient need to be transferred and bleeding has not been controlled kneel on the stretcher and maintain external manual aortic compression using the weight of your trunk.

Knee aortic compression is an option if you are alone or if the compression period will be prolonged.

The entire team should be trained so that person performing compression can be relieved if needed.

So uterine massage and aortic compression are very effective and inexpensive measures which when used timely and judiciously during the golden hour will help in saving precious lives of mothers.

SUGGESTED READING

1. ACOG practice bulletin Number 183 October 2017.
2. Bohren MA, Lorencatto F, Coomarasamy A, Althabe F, Devall AJ, Evans C, et al. Formative research to design an implementation strategy for a postpartum hemorrhage initial response treatment bundle (E-MOTIVE): study protocol. Reprod Health. 2021;18(1):149.
3. Escobar MF, Nassar AH, Theron G, Barnea ER, Nicholson W, Ramasauskaite D, et al. FIGO recommendations on the management of postpartum haemorrhage 2022. Int J Gynecol Obstet. 2022;157(Suppl. 1):3-50
4. Federation of Obstetrics and Gynecological Society of India. (2022). PPH Prevention and Management: Updated PPH Guidelines 2022 [online] Available from HYPERLINK "https://www.fogsi.org/wp-content/uploads/tog/pph%20 prevention-and-%20management-updated-sept-2022.pdf "https://www.fogsi.

org/wp-content/uploads/tog/pph prevention-and- management-updated-sept-2022.pdf [Last accessed December, 2025].

5. Mavrides E, Allard S, Chandraharan E, Green L, Hunt BJ, Riris S, et al. Prevention and Management Of PostpartumHaemorrhage: Green-top Guideline No. 52. BJOG An Int J Obstet Gynaecol. 2017;124(5):e106-49.
6. National Institutes of Health (NIH) | (.gov) https://pubmed.ncbi.nlm.nih.gov › ... by RC Pacagnella. 2022.
7. Patel, M. Postpartum Hemorrhage: Enhancing Outcomes for Mothers by Effective Management. J Obstet Gynecol India. 2024;74:191-5.
8. Resar R, Griffin FA, Haraden C, Nolan TW. Using Care Bundles to Improve Health Care Quality. IHI Innovation Series white paper. Cambridge, MA: Institute for Healthcare Improvement; 2012.
9. World Health Organization. WHO recommendations on the assessment of postpartum blood loss and use of a treatment bundle for postpartum haemorrhage. Geneva: WHO; 2023.

18 CHAPTER

Internal Iliac Artery Ligation in Postpartum Hemorrhage

Chandrakala Maran

INTRODUCTION

Internal iliac artery (IIA) is a branch of the common iliac artery (CIA) which is a branch of the Abdominal aorta. The Uterine artery is a branch of the Anterior division of IIA.

Internal iliac artery ligation (IIAL) essentially means ligation of its anterior division performed with a purpose of reducing blood flow to the Pelvic structures including the Uterus. IIA ligation to control intractable pelvic hemorrhage has been described by Kelly for the first time in 1893 for a cervical carcinoma case. Mengert and Burchel later popularized the procedure.

MECHANISM OF HEMOSTASIS

Bilateral IIAL reduces the pelvic arterial blood flow by 49% and pulse pressure by 85% mean arterial pressure by 25–50%. The ligation thereby converts arterial system into venous system leading to stable clot formation thus enabling hemostasis.

This helps to slow or stop hemorrhage while preserving blood flow via collateral circulation.

BRANCHES OF IIA

See **Flowchart 1**.

INDICATIONS

IIAL is a lifesaving procedure done in the following situations:

Following vaginal delivery:

- In Uterine atony where medical management, Balloon tamponades, Suction Cannula's, Compression sutures, Low and High Ligation of Uterine Arteries have failed.
- In Traumatic PPH with supralevator hematomas, cervical tears which have extended upwards causing Large Broad ligament hematomas

Flowchart 1: Branches of IIA.

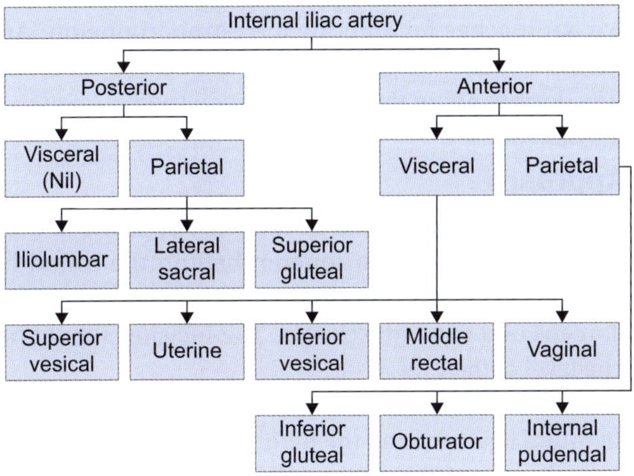

During cesarean sections:

- *Placenta accreta Spectrum:* Either prophylactic or Therapeutic IIAL is donc
- Extension of the lateral ends of caesarean incision with retracted uterine arteries and broad ligament hematomas

Other obstetric indications:

- Uterine rupture
- Nontubal ectopic pregnancies—cervical, interstitial, isthmic, and cesarean scar pregnancies

PREREQUISITES FOR IIAL

- Hemodynamically stable mother with near normal or normal coagulation profile
- Accessibility to blood and blood components
- Obstetrician or Surgeon skilled in IIAL
- Accessibility to a vascular surgeon
- Experienced anesthetist, operation theatre staff and special instruments.

PROCEDURE

Transperitoneal Approach

Transperitoneal approach is usually practiced.

Step 1: Entry into the Abdominal Cavity

Depending on clinical scenarios and expertise of the surgeon, a midline or transverse laparotomy or laparoscopy is performed. Midline laparotomy is preferred for Obstetric emergencies.

Step 2: Entry into Retroperitoneum

There are two approaches for entering the retroperitoneum: Anterior and Posterior. Surgeon based on his experience and his assessment of the pelvic anatomy decides about the appropriate method.

Anterior Approach

When the uterus is present it should be retracted opposite to the peritoneal incision for proper exposure. Peritoneum behind the round ligament at the junction of medial one-third and lateral two-third, is lifted with two long artery forceps and cut with scissors. The incision should be extended cranially to the level of the CIA.

When uterus is already removed, insert the scissors in between the cut ligated end of round ligament and the tubo-ovarian pedicle and cut upwards along the paracolic gutter **(Figs. 1A and B)**.

Step 3: Identification of the CIA Bifurcation

The psoas muscle is identified under the peritoneal incision with genito-femoral nerve coursing over it.

External iliac artery (EIA) runs along the medial border of psoas muscle and can be traced up to identify the CIA.

Step 4: Recognize External and Internal Iliac Arteries

The dissection should then progress in a cranio-caudal direction to track the course of the CIA and to prevent injury to underlying veins. The EIA and IIA should become visible, forming a " tripod" structure, with the ureter located medially and the EIA positioned laterally. The structure in the middle should be the IIA. To enhance certainty just before ligation, palpation of the bounding pulse over the arteries is recommended. The IIA typically follows an inferior and medial course, whereas the EIA has a slightly superior course just before entering the femoral ring **(Fig. 2)**.

Step 5: Lateral Pararectal Space Development

With dissection of Latzko's space, the ureter is retracted medially. It also offers sufficient space for the procedure.

Step 6: Site of Ligation of IIA

The IIA is approximately 4 cm in length before it divides into anterior and posterior branches The site of ligation is a point immediately after the IIA gives off its posterior division which is 3–4 cm after the origin of IIA from the CIA.

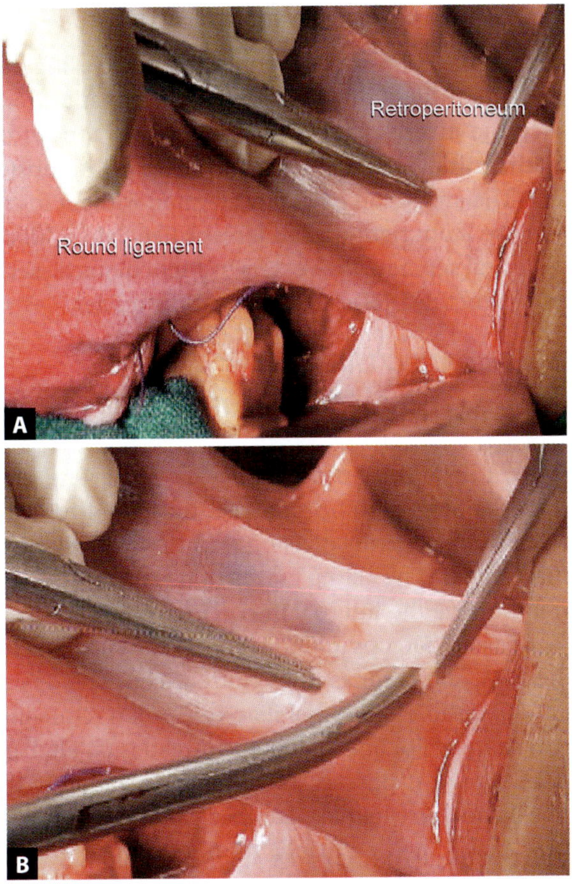

Figs. 1A and B: Step 2: Entry into retroperitoneum.

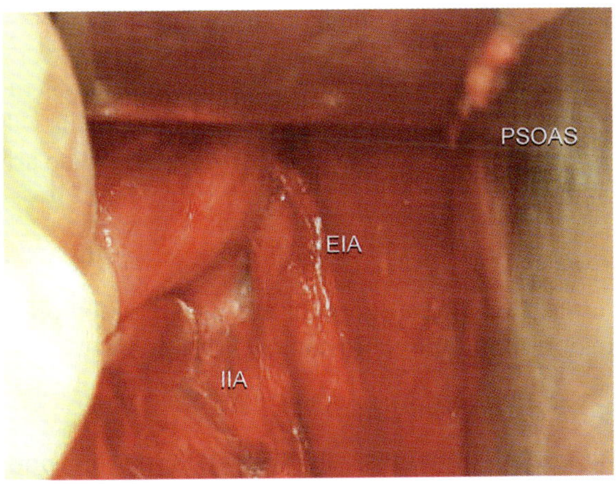

Fig. 2: Step 4: Recognize external and internal iliac arteries.

Step 7: Dissection of the Covering Sheath

Careful and gentle dissection of the fascial sheath enclosing the IIA is done at the proposed site of ligation. This step is the most critical part of the procedure since the artery often firmly adheres to the underlying vein. Clearing the adventitia of the artery may help to identify the correct dissection plane. The artery can be gently elevated without injuring the vein. It is advisable to use blunt right-angled forceps like Lahey, Mixter forceps or aneurysm needle and separate the vessels by meticulous dissection. A gap is made on either side of the artery gently to pass the mixter.

Step 8: Internal Iliac Artery Ligation

Absorbable Suture material Vicryl no 1-2 is doubled up and held with the tip of a mixter.

The instrument should be passed beneath the artery, approximately 3–4 cm below the bifurcation, from lateral to medial in order to ensure the ligation of only the anterior division and to avoid iatrogenic injury to the external iliac vessels. The clamp grazes transversely across the posterior wall of the artery to save the internal iliac vein posterior to it. The thread is grasped by a long artery forceps and the mixter/right angled clamp is gently removed in the same direction as it was introduced. The tips of the instrument should not point to the internal iliac vein when removing the forceps between the artery and vein. The loop of the thread is divided and the suture is tied. A double thread is passed so that if the accidently thread breaks during tying, we do not have to make another pass under the artery.

The ligatures should be tied firmly in order to avoid transection of the artery. An alternative technique is to use surgical clips to ligate the IIA, which eliminates the need for circumferential dissection, thereby reducing the chances of injury to the Iliac vein **(Figs. 3A and B)**.

Posterior Approach

The retroperitoneum may be opened 2-3 cm below and 2–3 cm lateral to the lateral end of upper border of the sacral promontory. This will open at the bifurcation of common iliac into external and internal iliac arteries. Rest of steps are the same.

Step 9: Palpation of Femoral Artery

Immediately after IIAL, the pulsation of the ipsilateral femoral artery within the inguinal region should be confirmed by palpation.

Step 10: Closure of Peritoneum

After ensuring complete hemostasis the peritoneal incision is closed in continuous manner with polyglycolic acid 2-0 or chromic catgut 2-0. with an abdominal drain.

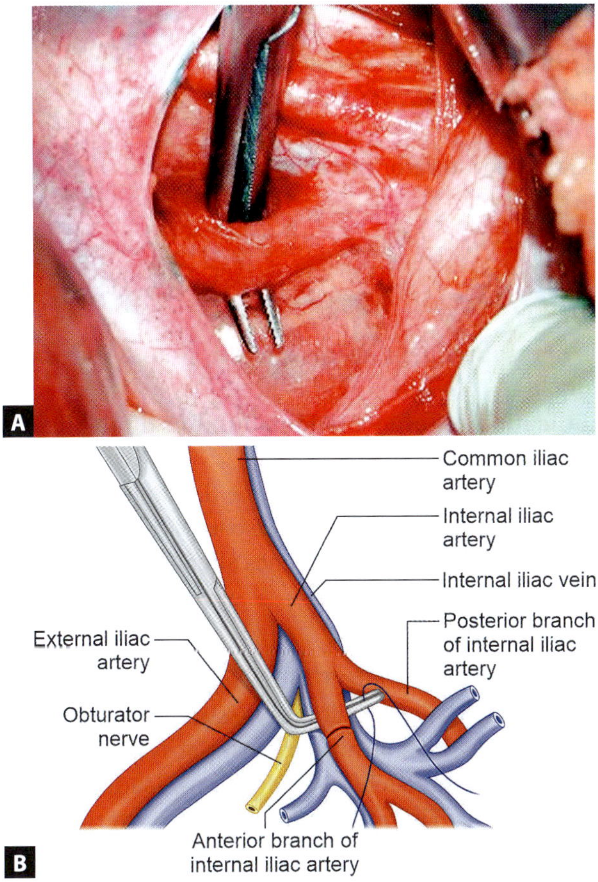

Figs. 3A and B: Step 8: Internal iliac artery ligation.

Extraperitoneal Approach for IIAL

The vessels supplying the pelvis and lower extremities are completely retroperitoneal. The parietal peritoneum is not incised, but reflected away from the midline along with the viscera.

- The area between the rectus muscle and peritoneum should be dissected
- The obliterated umbilical artery is identified and dissected downwards and laterally to track the internal iliac arteries.
- Dissection of the IIA upwards leads to the anterior division which is free and not as fixed as the posterior division.

COMPLICATIONS

Good knowledge of surgical anatomy, appropriate usage of surgical and hemostatic tools, and adherence to basic safety principles are precautions for reducing the incidence of complications and their severity.

Intraoperative

- Injury to external and internal iliac veins
- Accidental ligation of EIA or CIA
- Injury to ureter
- Rarely, injury to obturator nerve, truncus lumbosacralis, or the sciatic nerve
- EIA spasm and thrombosis

Postoperative

- Ischemia and subsequent necrosis of the gluteus maximus and pelvic visceral organs.
- Hip claudication, Atonic bladder, lumbosacral plexopathies and impotence.

Therefore, it is crucial that ligation of the IIA should be performed distal to its posterior division. Fortunately, these complications are rare due to the extensive collateral circulation in the pelvis after ligation.

Hemodynamics after IIAL

The primary hemodynamic effect following bilateral IIA ligation is the nearly complete elimination of blood pressure in small arteries distal to the ligation, effectively transforming the arterial system into a venous one. As a result, a hemostatic mechanism develops, leading to the formation and retention of clots. The pulse pressure and arterial blood pressure distal to the ligation decrease by 85% (with bilateral IIA ligation) and 25% (bilateral IIA ligation), respectively. Therefore, bilateral IIA ligation is more effective than unilateral ligation.

FERTILITY AND PREGNANCY OUTCOMES FOLLOWING IIAL

IIAL does not impair subsequent fertility and pregnancy outcomes probably due to good collateral circulation. Menses return normally, pregnancies occur and reach term without intrauterine growth restriction suggesting adequate blood supply. Nizard et al. reported a series of pregnancies following IIA ligation, with normal pregnancy outcomes and fertility among their population. Several other studies have reiterated the same outcome.

RECOMMENDATIONS

- IIAL should be performed by an experienced gynecologist or surgeon with enhanced knowledge of the anatomy of the pelvis.
- In situations with severe bleeding and hypovolemic shock, IIAL should be completed in less than 10 min.

- IIAL should be performed distal to the origin of the posterior division of the IIA
- Bilateral IIAL should be preferred.
- IIAL has to be considered prior to Obstetric Hysterectomy for women who desire fertility

CONCLUSION

IIAL is a critical and lifesaving procedure in cases of severe unexpected hemorrhage in obstetrics and gynecology. Its success relies on the expertise and skill of the surgeon. Therefore it should be integrated into obstetrics and gynecology postgraduate training programs itself.

SUGGESTED READING

1. B-Lynch C, Keith LG, Campbell WB. Internal iliac (hypogastric) artery ligation. In: B-Lynch C, Keith LG, Lalonde AB, Karosmi M (Eds). A Textbook of Postpartum Hemorrhage A Comprehensive Guide to Evaluation, Management and Surgical Intervention. 1st ed. Sapiens Publishing; London, UK: 2006. pp. 299-307.
2. B-Lynch C, Keith LG, Campbell WB. Internal iliac (hypogastric) artery ligation. In: B-Lynch C, Keith LG, Lalonde AB, Karosmi M (Eds). A Textbook of Postpartum Hemorrhage A Comprehensive Guide to Evaluation, Management and Surgical Intervention. 1st ed. Sapiens Publishing; London, UK: 2006. pp. 299-307.
3. Burchell RC. Physiology of internal iliac artery ligation. J Obstet Gynaecol Br Commonw. 1968;75:642-51.
4. Domingo S, Perales-Puchalt A, Soler I, Marcos B, Tamarit G, Pellicer A. Clinical outcome, fertility and uterine artery Doppler scans in women with obstetric bilateral internal iliac artery ligation or embolisation. J Obstet Gynaecol. 2013;33:701-4.
5. Kelly HA. Ligation of internal iliac arteries for hemorrhage in hysterectomy for carcinoma uteri. Bull Johns Hopkins Hosp. 1894;5:53.
6. Kostov S, Kornovski Y, Watrowski R, Slavchev S, Ivanova Y, Yordanov A. Internal Iliac Artery Ligation in Obstetrics and Gynecology: Surgical Anatomy and Surgical Considerations. Clin Pract. 2023;14(1):32-51.
7. Nabhan AE, AbdelQadir YH, Abdelghafar YA, Kashbour MO, Salem N, Abdelkhalek AN, et al. Therapeutic effect of Internal iliac artery ligation and uterine artery ligation techniques for bleeding control in placenta accreta spectrum patients: A meta-analysis of 795 patients. Front Surg. 2022;9: 983297.
8. Nizard J, Barrinque L, Frydman R, Fernandez H. Fertility and pregnancy outcomes following hypogastric artery ligation for severe post-partum haemorrhage. Hum Reprod. 2003;18:844-8.
9. Pai HD, Saxena M, Khadilkar S, Pandey A, Puri M. (2022). FOGSI FOCUS on Life Saving Emergency Obstetric Surgeries. [online] Available from https://fogsi.org/wp-content/uploads/fogsi-focus/FOGSI-Focus-Life-Saving-Emergency-Obstetric-Surgeries-2023.pdf [Last accessed December, 2025].

10. Raba G, Baran P. Hemodynamic parameters following bilateral internal iliac arteries ligation as a treatment of intrapartum hemorrhage. Ginekol. Pol. 2009; 80:179-83.
11. Raba G. Small invasive technique of Internal Iliac Artery ligation for postpartum haemorrhage. Ginekol Pol. 2020;91:29-31.
12. Sanders AP, Hobson SR, Kobylianskii A, Papillon Smith J, Allen L, Windrim R, et al. Internal iliac artery ligation-a contemporary simplified approach. Am J Obstet Gynecol. 2021;225:339.

19 CHAPTER

Nonpneumatic Antishock Garment in Obstetric Hemorrhage

Kirtan M Vyas, Munjal J Pandya

INTRODUCTION

Postpartum hemorrhage causes many maternal deaths in low and middle income countries. Globally PPH is the commonest cause of maternal deaths accounting for 25% of maternal mortality. The estimated prevalence of PPH varies from 2 to 11% of pregnancies. When defined by a blood loss of ≥500 mL, its prevalence varies from 10.5 to 26% in Africa, from 2.6 to 8% in Asia, from 6.3 to 13% in North America and Europe, and from 8 to 8.9% in Latin America. Postpartum hemorrhage continues to be a major cause of maternal mortality also in India. The reported incidence of PPH ranges from 2 to 4% after vaginal and 6% after cesarean delivery. Overall, it accounts for approximately 19.9% of maternal mortality in India which amounts to 78,000–117,000 deaths annually.

The nonpneumatic antishock garment helps you stabilize a woman with severe bleeding. It reduces blood loss and protects vital organ perfusion. It works as a temporizing device until you complete resuscitation and definitive procedures. Nonpneumatic antishock garment is a washable, low-weight, reusable compression suit made of neoprene. It consists of nine segments (three for each leg, one for pelvis, and one double segment for abdomen) which close tightly around legs, abdomen, and pelvis with Velcro **(Fig. 1)**.

MECHANISM OF ACTION

NASG exerts a circumferential pressure (usually up to 20–40 mm Hg) on blood vessels in legs, pelvis, and abdomen thereby decreasing blood flow in these vessels with a resultant improvement in blood circulation to more vital organs such as the brain, lungs, and heart. It also serves to reduce blood loss from the uterus by decreasing the uterine blood flow through compression of internal iliac artery. It allows access to perineal region and thus vaginal procedures can be performed easily without removing the suit. If any surgical access is needed, the segment which is applied at abdomen can be conveniently removed too. It is relatively cheap and easy to apply. Mere one hour of training is enough to educate nurses and primary care provides about its use. It does not exert pressure greater than 70 mm Hg and

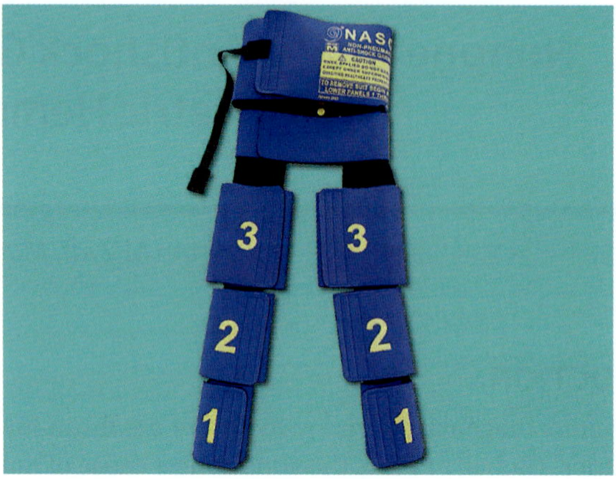

Fig. 1: NASG.

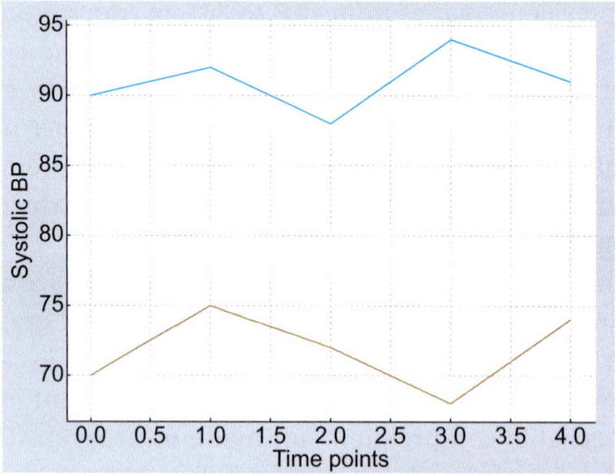

Fig. 2: Hemodynamic effects of NASG.

TABLE 1: NASG segment pressures.

Segment	*Approximate pressure*
Leg segments	20–25 mm Hg
Pelvic segment	30 mm Hg
Abdominal segment	35–40 mm Hg

thus there is no risk of ischemia of extremities or compartment syndrome **(Fig. 2 and Table 1)**.

APPLICATION

Place the woman flat. Apply lower segments first. Progress upward. Close the abdominal segment last. Check blood pressure every ten minutes.

Removal

Remove the abdominal segment last. Remove segments one by one in a monitored setting. Watch for recurrent hypotension.

HISTORY OF ANTISHOCK GARMENTS

The antishock garments were probably first used in 1900 when George Crile developed an inflatable pressure suit to maintain blood pressure during surgery.

In the 1970s, it underwent further modification into a half suit called military antishock trousers (MAST) or pneumatic antishock garment (PASG) and was used to control shock due to lower body hemorrhage. In the 1990s, its use was recommended by the American College of Obstetrics and Gynecology, which was subsequently revoked. Later, NASG was developed and first used in Pakistan as a temporary measure to improve blood flow to vital organs in PPH while waiting for more definitive treatment.

INDICATIONS

- Severe postpartum hemorrhage with systolic blood pressure less than 90 mm Hg
- Ongoing shock
- Referral or transport delays
- Limited access to blood products

CONTRAINDICATIONS

- Heart failure
- Pulmonary edema
- Acute cardiac disease
- Viable intrauterine pregnancy before delivery
- Severe abdominal trauma

BENEFITS

Studies report lower mortality. Blood loss reduces by 300 to 600 mL in several programs. Time to reach definitive care reduces because the woman stabilizes faster. NASG significantly reduced time to shock reversal. This is Important for preventing organ failure and minimizing transfusion needs. Therefore, it is found beneficial even when definitive hospital care is delayed.

Initial Evidence was found out in 2002 in which NASG was used in 6 women with severe PPH; 2 were pulseless. Dramatic improvement was noted in MAP and general condition. Bleeding stopped while NASG remained in place. But they recommended RCTs for further validation.

Severe hemorrhage study was carried out in Egypt and Nigeria in which 263 women were enrolled in study: 159 were subjected to NASG and 104 were controls. 64% decrease in median blood loss was recorded (740 → 250 mL). There were fewer deaths and morbidities and therefore combined outcome was significantly better (RR 0.28). This supported NASG effectiveness in severe cases.

Another study enrolled 854 women: 511 with NASG and reported 50% reduction in blood loss ($p < 0.0001$). There was also significant reduction in hysterectomies (RR 0.44), severe morbidity and mortality combined (RR 0.32) and maternal mortality (RR 0.35).

One interesting large multicountry study involving 1,442 women was caried out and published in 2013 with 835 NASG and 607 control. Mean blood loss reduced from 444 to 240 mL with maternal mortality reduced from 6.3% → 3.5% (RR 0.56) and severe morbidity reduced from 3.7% → 0.7% (RR 0.20). Most importantly, emergency hysterectomy reduced from 8.9% → 4%.

One real world Study was carried out in Tanzania in which 410 women with PPH and shock were subjected to be applied NASG during transport by trained workers. They noticed 67% reduction in case fatality rate (RR 0.33) and this highlighted effectiveness in pre-hospital settings.

FIGO RECOMMENDATIONS

Use NASG as temporary measure for:

- *Primary care or transport:* PPH >500 mL or SBP <100 or PR >100
- *Higher centers:* PPH >1,000 mL or SBP <90 or PR>110
- Apply from ankles upward
- Keep NASG in place until bleeding <25–50 mL/hour or source identified **(Table 2)**

FOGSI RECOMMENDATIONS

Use NASG:

- Where hemorrhage plays large role in maternal mortality
- Must address transportation delays and blood availability issues
- Training recommended for all healthcare providers involved in obstetric care
- Should be available at all healthcare levels including ambulances.

TABLE 2: Clinical outcomes with and without NASG.

Outcome	*Standard Care*	*NASG*
Mean blood loss	1,200 mL	700 mL
Transfusion need	65 percent	35 percent
Mortality	8 percent	4 percent

MESSAGE BOX

- Observational evidence strongly supports NASG in reducing blood loss and morbidity.
- RCT evidence is less conclusive but shows faster shock reversal.
- It is useful as temporary, life-saving adjunct, not stand-alone treatment.
- Future high-quality RCTs are needed to make it a more popular measure.

SUGGESTED READING

1. Abou Zahr C. Global burden of maternal death and disability. Br Med Bull. 2003;67:1-11.
2. ACOS. American College of Surgeons, Committee on Trauma. Advanced Trauma Life Support Manual. Chicago: American College of Surgeons; 1992.
3. Amy JJ. Severe Postpartum Hemorrhage: A Rational Approach. Natl Med J India. 1998;11(2):86-8.
4. Calvert C, Thomas SL, Ronsmans C, Wagner KS, Adler AJ, Filippi V. Identifying regional variation in the prevalence of postpartum haemorrhage: a systematic review and meta-analysis. PLoS One. 2012;7(7):e41114.
5. Carroli G, Cuesta C, Abalos E, Gulmezoglu AM. Epidemiology of postpartum haemorrhage: a systematic review. Best Pract Res Clin Obstet Gynaecol. 2008; 22(6):999-1012.
6. Cutler BS, Daggett WM. Application of the 'G-suit' to the control of hemorrhage in massive trauma. Ann Surg. 1971;173(4):511-4.
7. Hensleigh PA. Anti-shock garment provides resuscitation and haemostasis for obstetric haemorrhage. Br J Obstet Gynecol. 2002;109(12):1377-84.
8. Kumar N. Postpartum Hemorrhage; a Major Killer of Woman: Review of Current Scenario. Obstet Gynecol Inter J. 2016;4(4):00116.
9. Miller S, Bergel EF, El Ayadi AM, Gibbons L, Butrick EA, Magwali T, et al. Non-Pneumatic Anti-Shock Garment (NASG), a First-Aid Device to Decrease Maternal Mortality from Obstetric Hemorrhage: A Cluster Randomized Trial. PLoS One. 2013;8(10):e76477.
10. Miller S, Fathalla MM, Ojengbede OA, Camlin C, Mourad-Youssif M, Morhason-Bello IO, et al. Obstetric hemorrhage and shock management: using the low technology Non-pneumatic Anti Shock Garment in Nigerian and Egyptian tertiary care facilities. BMC Pregnancy Childbirth. 2010;10:64.
11. Miller S, Turan JM, Ojengbede A, Ojengbede O, Fathalla M, Morhason-Bello IO, et al. The pilot study of non-pneumatic anti-shock garment (NASG) in women with severe obstetric hemorrhage: Combined results from Egypt and Nigeria. Inter J Gynecol Obstet. 2006;94(Suppl 2):s154-6.
12. Ojengbede OA, Morhason-Bello IO, Galadanci H, Meyer C, Nsima D, Camlin C, et al. Assessing the role of the non-pneumatic anti-shock garment in reducing mortality from postpartum hemorrhage in Nigeria. Gynecol Obstet Invest. 2011;71(1):66-72.
13. Pileggi-Castro C, Nogueira-Pileggi V, Tunçalp Ö, Oladapo OT, Vogel JP, Souza JP. Non-pneumatic anti shock garment for improving maternal survival following severe postpartum haemorrhage: a systematic review. Reprod Health. 2015;12:28.

14. Sharma J, Negandhi P, Das AM, Sethy G, Neogi SB, Ali SH. Using nonpneumatic anti-shock garment for postpartum hemorrhage management and referral at the public health facilities: A pilot study in two districts of Bihar. Ind J Public Health. 2016;60:316-22.
15. Sutherland T, Downing J, Miller S, Bishai DM, Butrick E, Fathalla MM, et al. Use of the non-pneumatic anti shock garment (NASG) for life-threatening obstetric hemorrhage: a cost-effectiveness analysis in Egypt and Nigeria. PLoS One. 2013;8(4):e62282.
16. Vahedi M, Ayuyao A, Parsa MH, Freeman HP. Pneumatic Antishock Garment-Associated Compartment Syndrome in Uninjured Lower Extremities. J Trauma Acute Care Surg. 1995;384(4):616-8.

20 CHAPTER

Balloon Tamponade in Management of Postpartum Hemorrhage

Ashish Narendra Zarariya

INTRODUCTION

WHO guidelines for management of PPH had strongly suggested use of balloon tamponade. Uterine balloon tamponade is recommended for the treatment of postpartum hemorrhage due to uterine atony after vaginal birth in women who do not respond to standard first-line treatment, provided the following conditions are met:

- Immediate recourse to surgical intervention and access to blood products is possible if needed.
- A primary postpartum hemorrhage first-line treatment protocol (including the use of uterotonics, tranexamic acid, intravenous fluids) is available and routinely implemented.
- Other causes of postpartum hemorrhage (retained placental tissue, trauma) can be reasonably excluded.
- The procedure is performed by health personnel who are trained and skilled in the management of postpartum hemorrhage, including the use of uterine balloon tamponade.
- Maternal condition can be regularly and adequately monitored for prompt identification of any signs of deterioration.

While there is insufficient evidence from randomized trials conducted in low-resource settings to assess the benefits and potential harms of uterine balloon tamponade when used for PPH treatment, several observational studies suggest a substantial reduction in the risk of maternal morbidity after uterine balloon tamponade use. It is unclear whether this disparity in findings reflects study design, balloon type or access to other essential components of PPH care. The impact of uterine balloon tamponade for PPH treatment on health equity and cost is likely to vary according to uterine balloon tamponade designs (low-cost improvised or purpose-designed devices versus expensive purpose-designed devices). In contexts where standard PPH treatment protocols are available and implemented, uterine balloon tamponade use for PPH treatment is probably feasible and acceptable to women and providers.

MECHANISM OF ACTION OF BALLOON TAMPONADE

UBT works on 2 main principles.

1. It exerts inward to outward pressure which in high pressure low volume balloons becomes sometimes greater than the systemic arterial pressure (like in Bakri Balloon), while in high volume low pressure balloon inward to outward pressure over uterine wall never goes beyond venous pressure (like in Burkes ESM-UBT Balloon).
2. UBT also exerts hydrostatic pressure which exerts pressure on uterine arteries thereby reducing bleeding.

TYPES OF UBT

Historically different types of improvised balloons were in use **(Figs. 1A and B)**.

There is no standard classification systems, but depending on their action UBT is mainly divided into 3 main categories as explained above:

1. *High pressure low volume balloon:* They are purpose designed devices hence expensive Examples is Bakri Balloon.
2. *High volume low pressure balloon:* They are mostly low cost improvised devices. Example is Burkes Balloon.
3. *Dynamic balloon:* They are designed so as to fit in atonic uterus. Distending fluid goes inside the balloon with gravity. As uterine tone is achieved fluid automatically goes back in container. Example is Ellavi Balloon.

We were part of ESM UBT project (Every Second Matter—UBT) since 2018. We had experience of using all these 3 types of balloon. Every Balloon had its own advantage and disadvantages, but we found these high volume low pressure types of Burkes balloon **(Fig. 2)** more useful over others because of following reasons.

- Low cost
- *Ease of use:* With little training even Nursing staff can use it in life saving scenarios.
- *Rigid catheter and retention balloon:* Prevents it from coming out with rapid flowing blood.
- Special one way valve with easy fitted syringe - help introducing water at an rapid rate just like using an Hysteromat in hysteroscopy.

ESM UBT (Burkes Balloon) Complete Kit

- 2 condoms
- 2 0-rings
- 1 Foley catheter fitted with a one-way valve
- A 60 mL syringe

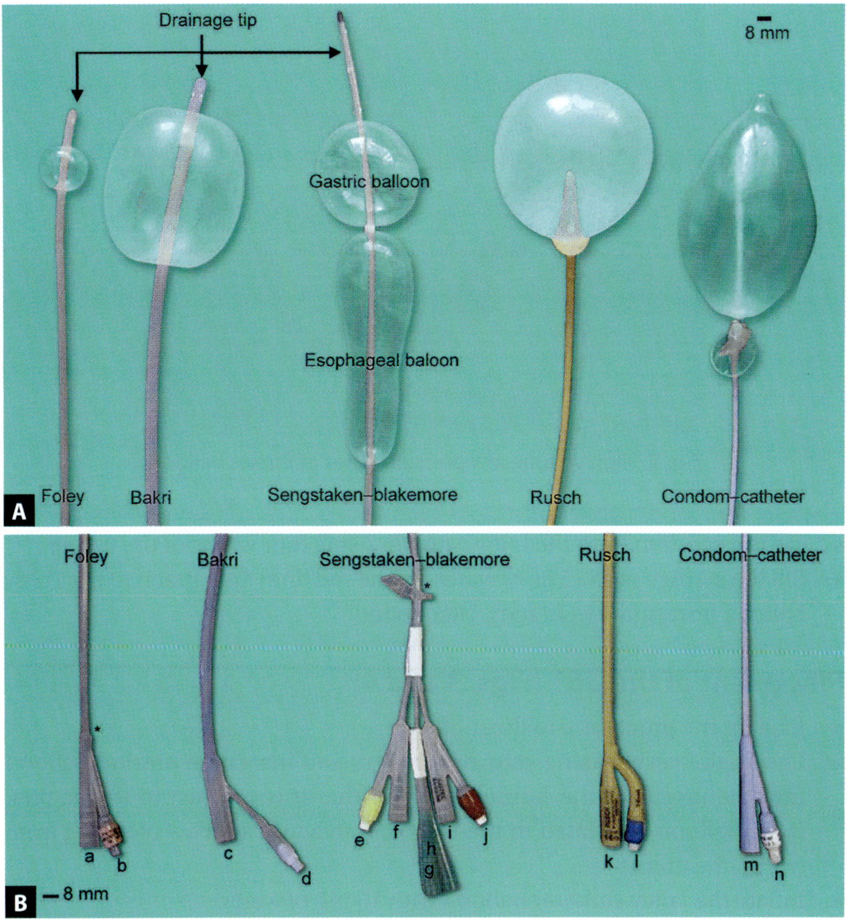

- b, d, e, f, i, j, k and m indicate insufflation portion of balloon
- a, c, g and h indicate drainage portion of uterine cavity
- l and n do not contribute to balloon tamponade or drainage. They inflate a balloon within the actual tamponade balloon
- There is no drainage of the uterine cavity when using the Rusch and condom catheter

Figs. 1A and B: Types of UBT.

- A leg attachment
- An instruction card
- A data card.

Assembly of the UBT

- Collect the already assembled ESM-UBT kit, a basin and clean water.
- Put on long clean gloves.
- Open the kit and place items on a clean surface.
- Unroll the condom. Place the Foley catheter half-way into the condom leaving the condom hanging loosely at the end of the foley.

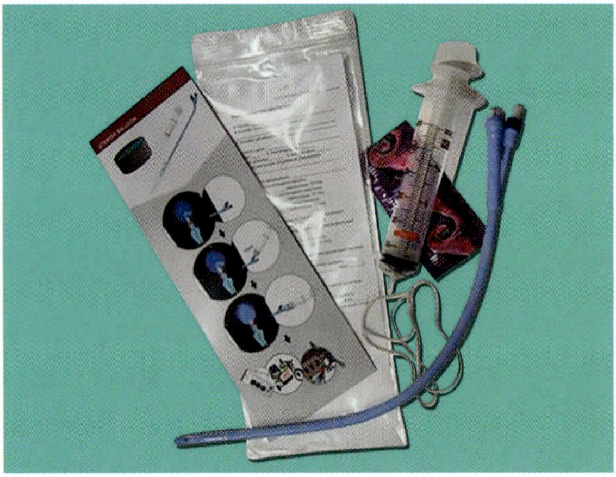

Fig. 2: High volume low pressure types of Burkes balloon.

- Tie the condom onto the foley catheter using four wraps of the 0-ring
- Fill the syringe with 15 cc of water (to the red line) and attach to the Foley balloon port (marked in red). "Red to red"

Placement of the UBT (Figs. 3 and 4)

- Explain the procedure to the mother.
- Locate the cervix using your two fingers and insert the uterine balloon into the uterus to the fundus. Be sure that it is not just in the vagina. If the balloon is inflated in the vagina, it may not address bleeding from within the uterus.
- Inflate the Foley catheter balloon with 15 mL of water.
- Inflate the condom balloon through the one-way valve using clean water at room temperature. Fill the balloon until the bleeding stops. This usually with 300–500 mL of water, but may require more as uterine sizes vary. Stop of increased resistance is felt and the bleeding has not stopped. Make sure the balloon is correctly placed. If so, look for other causes of bleeding.
- Continue to check to see that the UBT has not slipped into the vagina as it is filled.
- Secure the catheter on the thigh of the woman so it does not pull out with her movement.

After successful insertion of the UBT the mother is ready for careful observation or transfer to a referral facility.

- If no other procedures are need, the woman may be placed in recovery position.
- Give a prophylactic dose of broad-spectrum antibiotics such as IV/IM ceftriaxone.

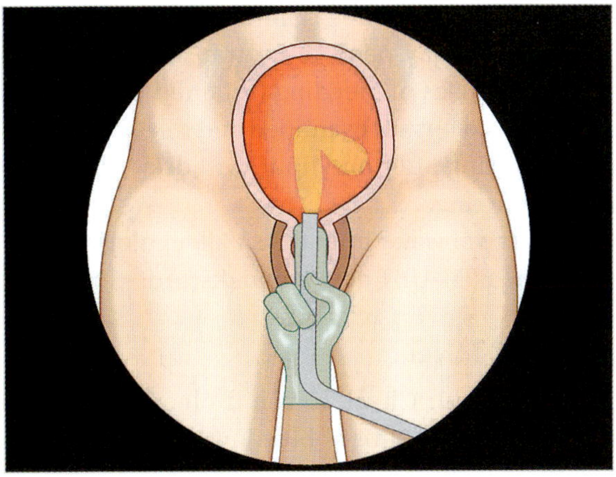

Fig. 3: Placement of the UBT.

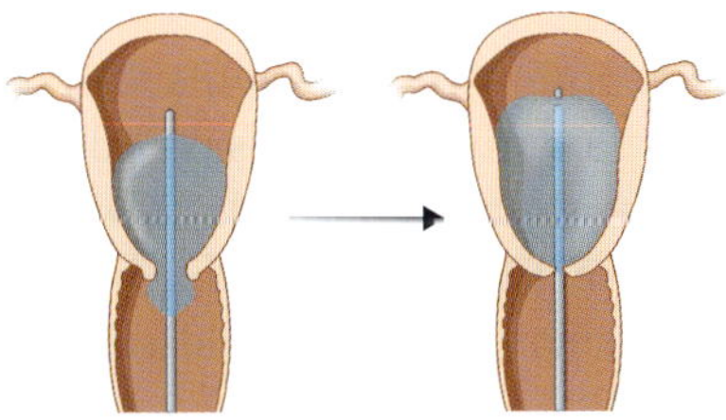

Fig. 4: Placement of the UBT.

- IV fluids and uterotonics should continue.
- Treat shock as indicated. Monitor urine output. (Should produce an average of more than 30 mL per hour of urine.).
- Monitor the mother's vitals and bleeding at least every 15 minutes for the first 2 hours and for longer if the mother is not yet stable. Then monitor every 4 hours.
- Teach the mother to inform you immediately if there is increased bleeding or if the balloon becomes dislodged.

Removal

The uterine balloon should stay in place for at least 6-24 hours. If a decision to transfer the mother is made, the balloon should not be removed before transfer.

- Explain the procedure to the mother
- Wash your hands and put on gloves.
- Remove 100 mL of water from the balloon through the one-way valve and observe closely for one hour to see if bleeding resumes.

- If significant bleeding resumes refill the balloon and re-examine the patient. The patient may need to be transferred to a higher level of care where other causes of bleeding (retained products, cervical tears, coagulopathy) can be further examined and treated.
- If there is no bleeding after one hour, withdraw all the water from the balloon using the syringe.
- Withdraw the 15 mL of water from the smaller Foley catheter balloon.
- Gently remove the ESM-UBT device and discard.

TROUBLE SHOOTING

- *If the balloon falls out:* Check to see if bleeding has resumed. If so, check the source and amount of bleeding. A new balloon may need to be placed. If there is no bleeding, observe the patient closely to be sure bleeding does not resume. You do not need to replace the balloon if there is no bleeding even if you are less than 6 hours from original placement.
- *If the patient is uncomfortable:* Patients usually have only minor cramping with the balloon in place. A small dose of an oral analgesic is reasonable to help with this if needed. If pain is severe, evaluate the patient. check for correct UBT placement, infection or other causes. Sometimes removing a small amount of fluid will help without resumption of bleeding

CONTRAINDICATIONS

- Uterine rupture
- Latex allergy (rare)
- Relative contraindications are cervical tears, chorioamnionitis, retained POCs, and cervical cancer. However in life-threatening conditions and in the absence of any other measures to stop bleeding in low resource settings UBT still can be helpful.

It should be used on every patient who meets criteria for the Response to Refractory Bleeding bundle, that is, bleeding does not stop with uterotonics, uterine message, and tranexamic acid.

What do you do after the UBT is placed?

- Give a prophylactic dose of broad-spectrum antibiotics such as IV/IM ceftriaxone
- IV fluids and uterotonics should continue.
- Treat shock as indicated. Monitor urine output. (Should produce an average of more than 30 mL per hour of urine.)
- Monitor the mother's vitals and bleeding at least every 15 minutes for the first 2 hours and for longer if the mother is not yet stable. Then monitor every 4 hours.

SUMMARY

UBT has high success rate for treating postpartum hemorrhage not responding to medical management, its safe and cost effective in certain settings.

SUGGESTED READING

1. Burke TF, Shivkumar PV, Priyadarshani P, Garg L, Conde-Agudelo A, Guha M. Impact of the introduction of a low- cost uterine balloon tamponade (ESM-UBT) device for managing severe postpartum hemorrhage in India: A comparative before- and- after study. Int J Gynaecol Obstet. 2022;159(2): 466-73.
2. Santhoshi D, Yaliwal RG, Patil N, Biradar A. (2025). Comparative Study of the Safety and Efficacy of a Prophylactic Insertion of Dr. Burke's Every Second Matters-Uterine Balloon Tamponade (ESM-UBT) With IM Oxytocin vs. Only IM Oxytocin for the Prevention of Atonic PPH: A Randomized Parallel Group Trial. [online] Available from https://assets.cureus.com/uploads/original_article/pdf/352730/20250511-305067-ma3ego.pdf [Last accessed December, 2025].
3. Vogel JP, Wilson AN, Scott N, Widmer M, Althabe F, Oladapo OT. Cost-effectiveness of uterine tamponade devices for the treatment of postpartum hemorrhage: A systematic review. Int J Gynaecol Obstet. 2020;151(3):333-340.
4. WHO guidelines of PPH https://doi.org/10.1016/S0140-6736(25)01639-3.

CHAPTER 21

Early Detection, Risk Stratification, and Nonclinical Components of Management of Postpartum Hemorrhage

Rajasi Kane Sengupta

INTRODUCTION

Postpartum hemorrhage (PPH) is the one of the leading direct causes of maternal mortality worldwide and in India, responsible for nearly one-quarter of maternal deaths. Most deaths are preventable through timely recognition, risk stratification, and organized facility-level response. Early detection and systematic risk stratification are key components of the WHO and FIGO recommendations for reducing PPH-related mortality. In India, national programs such as *LaQshya Labor Room Quality Improvement Initiative, Dakshata program, Janani Suraksha Yojana (JSY), Janani Shishu Suraksha Karyakram (JSSK), and Anemia Mukt Bharat (AMB)* strengthen the ecosystem for the timely identification and management of PPH. Non-clinical components—team readiness, standardized protocols, simulation drills, logistics, audits, and communication pathways—significantly improve outcomes when layered over clinical management strategies.

WHO defines primary PPH as blood loss ≥1,000 mL within 24 hours of birth, or any blood loss causing hemodynamic instability, irrespective of the measured volume. In Indian programs and peripheral settings, ≥500 mL after vaginal birth is often used as an operational trigger for action, to avoid delay.

EARLY DETECTION OF POSTPARTUM HEMORRHAGE

Definition

The WHO defines PPH as *≥1,000 mL blood loss within 24 hours or any blood loss causing hemodynamic instability*, regardless of volume. Indian facilities, particularly primary and secondary centers, continue to use ≥500 mL after vaginal birth as a practical marker for early response **(Table 1)**.

- *Primary PPH*—blood loss exceeding 500 mL in a vaginal delivery or 1,000 mL in a caesarean section, or any loss causing shock within 24 hours of delivery.
- *Severe PPH*—blood loss more than 1,000 mL, need for transfusion, or hemodynamic compromise.
- *Secondary PPH*—bleeding occurring after 24 hours postpartum through 42 days or 6 weeks (till end of puerperium).

TABLE 1: Classification of postpartum hemorrhage.

Type	*Time frame*	*Definition*
Primary PPH	0–24 hours	Blood loss ≥500 mL vaginal or ≥1,000 mL operative
Severe PPH	Within 24 hours	≥1,000 mL or shock
Secondary PPH	24 hours–6 weeks	Abnormal/excess bleeding postpartum

Importance of Early Detection

Blood loss is underestimated by *50–80%*, delaying life-saving intervention. Delays in recognition and response ("three delays") are major contributors in Indian maternal death and near-miss audits.

COMPONENTS OF EARLY DETECTION

Quantification of Blood Loss

National programs including *Dakshata* and *LaQshya* mandate *routine quantification of blood loss (QBL) for all deliveries*, using calibrated drapes and gravimetric measurement. QBL > 350 mL in the first 10–15 minutes predicts severe PPH progression. Relying on visual estimation alone is not recommended.

Preferred Methods (also Promoted in Dakshata and LaQshya Labor Rooms)

- Use of calibrated under-buttock PPH drapes (e.g. BRASS-V).
- Gravimetric method:
  - Blood loss (mL) ≈ weight of soaked materials (g)—dry weight.
  - Volumetric measurement from suction jars.
  - Cumulative QBL charted every 15 minutes in the immediate postpartum period.

Early QBL ≥300–350 mL within 10–15 minutes alerts the team to impending severe PPH and triggers escalation.

Physiological Monitoring and Early Warning Scores

Modified Obstetric Early Warning System (MEOWS/MOEWS) charts are advised to detect early deterioration.

Parameters commonly tracked:

- Pulse rate, blood pressure (BP) trend
- Respiratory rate (RR)
- Oxygen saturation (SpO_2)
- Conscious level/mental status
- Urine output

Any single red-zone value or two yellow-zone values should prompt immediate clinical review and consideration of PPH or other obstetric emergencies. Deviation triggers a *"PPH Alert"* within LaQshya quality-assurance protocols.

Clinical Red Flags

See **Table 2**.

India-specific Programmatic Triggers

National initiatives such as Dakshata and LaQshya (Labor Room and Maternity OT Quality Improvement Initiative) integrate early detection of PPH into case sheets and checklists:

- Mandatory documentation of QBL for every delivery.
- MEOWS chart use in LaQshya labor rooms.
- Standard prompts for "PPH alert" when QBL ≥500 mL or physiological triggers appear.
- Checklist reminders for early use of uterotonics and tranexamic acid,
- as per WOMAN trial evidence.

Point-of-Care Testing

Although limited at peripheral centers, tertiary hospitals use:

- Lactate
- Base deficit
- TEG/ROTEM for early coagulopathy
- Rapid Hb estimation using digital devices (HemoCue)

GOI recommends availability under *FRU (First Referral Unit) strengthening policy*.

Role of Ultrasound

Ultrasound in PPH case is not diagnostic alone, but a decision-supportive tool.

TABLE 2: Clinical red flags.

Red flag	*Meaning*
HR >110/min	Early shock
Narrow pulse pressure	Compensatory vasoconstriction
• No uterine tone • Persistent vaginal bleeding despite uterotonics • Uterus soft, boggy or poorly contracted	Atony/trauma
Falling urine output	End-organ ischemia

It can be useful for identifying:

- Retained products
- Broad ligament hematoma
- Free fluid
- Poor uterine contraction

RISK STRATIFICATION FOR PPH

Risk stratification allows planning of place of delivery, level of care required and readiness for hemorrhage. Risk stratification aligns with WHO, FIGO, ACOG and is integrated into India's *Dakshata checklists, LaQshya case sheets, and High-Risk Pregnancy (HRP) tracking system.*

Antenatal Risk Factors

- Anemia (<10 g/dL)—high prevalence in India, addressed under *Anemia Mukt Bharat*
- Previous PPH
- Multiple pregnancy, polyhydramnios
- Grand multiparity
- Obesity
- Coagulopathies, thrombocytopenia
- Placenta previa or placenta accreta spectrum (PAS).
- Hypertensive disorders

Intrapartum Risk Factors (Table 3)

- Induction or augmentation with oxytocin
- Prolonged or obstructed labor
- Instrumental or operative delivery
- Cesarean section
- Chorioamnionitis and fever
- Precipitate labor
- Retained placenta or membranes

Risk category determines number of IV lines, blood cross-match requirements, need for consultant presence and OR stand-by.

RISK STRATIFICATION MODELS USED IN INDIA

WHO–FIGO Models

Low, Moderate, and High risk based on history and intrapartum events.

ACOG Levels

High-risk includes placenta previa/accreta, low platelets, severe anemia.

TABLE 3: Risk factors for PPH and facility level.

Practical risk categories (for use in labor room)	*Risk factors*	*Required facility level*
Low	• Singleton • Term • No comorbidity • No major antenatal/intrapartum risks	Any facility with SBA
Moderate	• Mild anemia • Induction • Prolonged labor • Multiple pregnancy	FRU/LaQshya facility
High	• Placenta previa • Severe anemia Hb <8 g/dL • Severe preeclampsia • Previous PPH • Thrombocytopenia • Major fibroids	CEmONC center
Very high	• PAS • Severe anemia • Complex cardiac disease • Coagulopathy	Tertiary center with ICU, LaQshya-certified CEmONC center with blood bank, interventional radiology or surgical backup if available

Government of India (GoI) HRP Score

- Integrated into Mother and Child Tracking System (MCTS)
- Red-flag patients to deliver only at FRU/CEmONC centers

LaQshya Color Coding

- *Green*—low risk
- *Yellow*—moderate
- *Red*—high risk requiring consultant-led delivery

Use of AI Models (Emerging)

Machine-learning tools incorporating:

- Labor curve patterns
- Vitals trends
- QBL trajectories
- Past obstetric history.

  These improve prediction accuracy over static scoring.

Translating Risk Stratification into Indian Labor Rooms

See **Table 4**.

Nonclinical Components of PPH Management

Non-clinical components often determine whether clinical actions can be implemented *within the "Golden 5–10 minutes"* of PPH response.

India has incorporated global standards into national programs such as *Dakshata, LaQshya, SBA (Skilled Birth Attendant), FRU strengthening, and Maternal Near-Miss Reviews.*

PROTOCOLS AND CHECKLISTS (TABLE 5)

National Standardized PPH Protocols

Aligned with WHO and FIGO guidelines, including:

- Early uterotonics
- TXA within 3 hours (WOMAN Trial)
- Stepwise escalation for atony, trauma, retained placenta, coagulopathy
- Massive transfusion protocol (MTP) activation

TABLE 4: Translating risk stratification into Indian labor rooms.

Risk group	*Recommended action (as per Dakshata/LaQshya)*
Low	Active management of third stage (AMTSL)
Moderate	Two IV lines, keep blood ready, staff readiness
High	Senior obstetrician-led delivery, massive transfusion protocol (MTP) readiness, ultrasound support
Very High (PAS, severe anemia)	Delivery in *CEmONC LaQshya-certified center*, OR standby, blood products immediately available

TABLE 5: Nonclinical preparedness components.

Component	*Examples in Indian context*	*Description*
Readiness	Protocols, kits, training	PPH cart, drugs, supplies, team roles, Dakshata/LaQshya checklists, SBA training
Recognition	Early detection	QBL, MEOWS charts, PPH alert triggers
Response	Timely management	Rapid uterotonics and TXA, balloon tamponade, MTP
Reporting	Audit and feedback	Documentation, handover, dashboards
Review		MDR, near-miss review (NMR), PPH dashboards, QI meetings

Dakshata Checklists

Cover:
- QBL
- PPH risk screening
- AMTSL
- Availability of uterotonics
- Team roles
- Documentation

LaQshya Labor Room Case Sheets

Include:
- PPH early-warning prompts
- Standardized charting
- Handover checklists
- Emergency trigger forms

PPH Emergency Carts

Mandated under *LaQshya certification* with:
- Oxytocin, tranexamic acid
- IV sets
- Balloon tamponade (CG balloon/simplified condom catheter)
- Suturing sets
- Crystalloid fluids
- Gloves, cannulas

THE 4 R'S OF PPH PREPAREDNESS (FIGO + INDIA ADOPTION)

- *Readiness*—PPH kits, checklists, simulation
- *Recognition*—QBL, MEOWS
- *Response*—timely uterotonics, TXA, balloon
- *Reporting*—maternal near-miss review committees

In India, these map to:
- *Readiness* → Dakshata checklists
- *Recognition* → LaQshya MOEWS
- *Response* → FRU-level PPH pathway
- *Reporting* → Maternal Death Review (MDR), Maternal Near-Miss Review (MNMR)

TEAM-BASED PREPAREDNESS

Role Allocation

Clear role definition is part of Dakshata training modules **(Table 6)**.

TABLE 6: Role allocation.

Team member	*Role*
Obstetrician	Leads clinical care
Senior resident	Executes stepwise algorithm
Junior resident	Assists procedures
Anesthetist	Airway, fluids, vasopressors
Nurse	QBL, drug preparation
Blood bank officer	Blood products
Runner	Logistics, communication

Simulation Drills

Simulation drills are required for *LaQshya certification*. Simulation reduces errors and improves coordination, They are conducted quarterly. The list of drills includes:
- Atonic PPH
- PPH during CS
- Balloon tamponade insertion
- MTP activation

COMMUNICATION SYSTEMS

Closed-loop Communication

Reinforced during SBA and Dakshata trainings.

PPH Alert Systems

Activated when:
- QBL ≥ 500 mL
- MEOWS triggers
- Sudden vital instability

Documentation

The LaQshya partograph and PPH sheets ensure:
- Timings of interventions
- QBL logs
- Transfer and referral notes

FACILITY-LEVEL PREPAREDNESS IN INDIA

LaQshya Labor Rooms

These feature:
- QR-coded checklists

- Dedicated emergency trolleys
- Clean, well-equipped labor rooms
- Real-time dashboard monitoring

FRU and CEmONC Strengthening

- Availability of C-section capability
- Blood storage centers
- Trained obstetricians and anesthesiologists

Blood Bank Readiness

Aligned with WHO and FIGO recommendations

- Massive transfusion protocol (MTP) flowchart displayed
- Immediate O-negative availability
- Cryoprecipitate and FFP availability

AUDITS AND QUALITY IMPROVEMENT

Maternal Death Review (MDR)

Used nationwide to identify systemic delays.

Maternal Near-Miss Review (MNMR)

Focuses on preventable factors—key to PPH improvement.

PPH Dashboards

LaQshya centers maintain:

- Number of PPH cases
- Interventions used
- Usage of TXA
- Balloon tamponade numbers
- Morbidity and near-miss cases

COMMUNITY AND PUBLIC HEALTH STRATEGIES (INDIA)

Anemia Mukt Bharat (AMB)

Reduces antenatal anemia, a major PPH risk factor.

JSY/JSSK Schemes

Improve institutional delivery rates and timely referral.

Referral Transport Systems

108/102 ambulance networks for rapid movement to FRU/CEmONC.

SBA Training

Ensures every ANM/Staff Nurse can:

- Perform AMTSL
- Give TXA
- Insert condom balloon
- Initiate PPH protocol

Standard Referral Pathways

Mandated by GOI for:

- Placenta previa/accreta
- Severe anemia
- HRP cases

DIGITAL HEALTH AND AI IN INDIA

- *HMIS and MCTS:* Track HRP and PPH data
- *AI-based prediction models* (pilot projects)
- *Digital partogram*
- *Wearable monitoring devices* in high-risk mothers

KEY TAKE-HOME MESSAGE

- Early detection through QBL, MEOWS, and vigilant clinical surveillance remains central to reducing maternal deaths from PPH.
- India's national initiatives—Dakshata, LaQshya, Anemia Mukt Bharat, FRU strengthening, and SBA training—integrate global standards into facility and community settings to improve preparedness and response.
- Risk stratification through antenatal HRP tracking and LaQshya color coding guides preparedness and appropriate facility-based delivery.
- Non-clinical components such as PPH kits, emergency drills, standardized checklists, rapid communication pathways, blood bank readiness, and robust audit systems are essential for timely action.
- The implementation of TXA within 3 hours, AMTSL, and the stepwise response protocol integrated in Dakshata further enhances outcomes.
- National quality-improvement programs strengthen system responsiveness.
- Audits and dashboards sustain continuous improvement.
- When these evidence-based, system-level strategies are consistently implemented, India can significantly reduce preventable maternal mortality due to PPH and achieve SDG-3 maternal health goals.

SUGGESTED READING

1. ACOG Practice Bulletin No. 183: Postpartum hemorrhage. Obstet Gynecol. 2017;130:e168-86.
2. American College of Obstetricians and Gynecologists. ACOG Practice Bulletin No. 183: Postpartum hemorrhage. Obstet Gynecol. 2017;130:e168-86.

3. FIGO guidelines: management of postpartum haemorrhage. Int J Gynaecol Obstet. 2012;119:119-26.
4. International Federation of Gynecology and Obstetrics. FIGO guidelines: management of postpartum haemorrhage. Int J Gynaecol Obstet. 2012;119: 119-26.
5. Kellie FJ, Wandabwa JN. Using Modified Obstetric Early Warning Score charts to detect early signs of deterioration. Int J Gynaecol Obstet. 2021;152(1):64-70.
6. Patel A, Goudar SS, Geller SE, Kodkany BS, Edlavitch SA, Wagh K, et al. Drape estimation vs visual assessment for blood loss after delivery: a randomized trial. Am J Obstet Gynecol. 2006;195(1):54-8.
7. Sentilhes L, Vayssière C, Deneux-Tharaux C, Aya AG, Bayoumeu F, Bonnet MP, et al. Postpartum hemorrhage: guidelines for clinical practice. J Gynecol Obstet Hum Reprod. 2020;49(8):101861.
8. Shakur-Still H, Medcalf KE, Novikova N. Implementation of tranexamic acid for postpartum haemorrhage: what do we know and what is needed? Int J Obstet Anesth. 2023;45:103211.
9. Sheldon WR, Blum J, Vogel JP, Souza JP, Gülmezoglu AM, Winikoff B; WHO Multicountry Survey on Maternal and Newborn Health Research Network. Postpartum haemorrhage management, risks, and maternal outcomes: findings from the WHO Multicountry Survey. BJOG. 2014;121 Suppl 1:5-13.
10. Weeks A. The prevention and treatment of postpartum haemorrhage: what do we know, and where do we go next? BJOG. 2015;122(2):202-10.
11. WOMAN Trial Collaborators. Effect of early tranexamic acid administration on mortality, hysterectomy, and other morbidities in women with postpartum haemorrhage (WOMAN): an international, randomized, double-blind, placebo-controlled trial. Lancet. 2017;389(10084):2105-16.
12. World Health Organization. WHO recommendations for the prevention and treatment of postpartum haemorrhage. Geneva: WHO; 2012.
13. World Health Organization. WHO recommendations for the prevention and treatment of postpartum haemorrhage. Geneva: WHO; 2012.

22 CHAPTER

Teamwork, Communication, and Record Maintenance in the Management of Postpartum Hemorrhage

Ashwin Rao

INTRODUCTION

Postpartum hemorrhage (PPH) remains the leading direct cause of maternal mortality globally, particularly in low- and middle-income countries like India. According to the World Health Organization (WHO), approximately *25% of maternal deaths* worldwide are due to PPH. In India, PPH accounts for *30–38% of maternal mortality*, with many of these deaths being preventable through timely and coordinated action.

Modern management of PPH has moved beyond reliance solely on clinical skills or protocols—it now necessitates *interdisciplinary teamwork*, *effective communication*, and *meticulous documentation*. The combination of these three pillars creates a system where early recognition, rapid response, and accountability are seamlessly integrated into maternal care.

This chapter comprehensively discusses the critical importance of teamwork, communication, and record maintenance in the management of PPH, contextualized to both *primary-level obstetric units* and *tertiary care hospitals*.

UNDERSTANDING PPH: SCOPE AND CLINICAL IMPLICATIONS

Postpartum hemorrhage is defined as *blood loss ≥500 mL after vaginal birth* or *≥1,000 mL after cesarean section*, occurring within 24 hours of delivery (primary PPH), or beyond 24 hours to 6 weeks postpartum (secondary PPH).

Clinical Classification

- *Minor PPH:* 500–1,000 mL with no signs of shock.
- *Major PPH:* >1,000 mL or any blood loss associated with hemodynamic instability.

Etiologies

The 4 Ts:

1. *Tone (70–80%):* Uterine atony.
2. *Tissue:* Retained placental tissue.

3. *Trauma:* Genital tract lacerations, uterine rupture.
4. *Thrombin:* Coagulopathy.

Each cause requires a different management pathway, and timely differentiation among these is only possible with *clear task delegation, rapid communication,* and *well-documented assessments.*

IMPORTANCE OF A MULTIDISCIPLINARY TEAM APPROACH IN PPH

Effective PPH management mandates involvement from:

- Obstetricians
- Anesthesiologists
- Nurses and midwives
- Blood bank staff
- Critical care teams (in severe cases)
- Support staff including attenders and ambulance services

Key Attributes of a PPH Response Team

- *Role clarity:* Everyone should know their responsibilities before, during, and after an obstetric emergency.
- *Shared mental model:* Team members must have a common understanding of the situation, expected outcomes, and steps to be taken.
- *Situational awareness:* Team leaders should monitor team performance and the patient's clinical status in real-time.

Example of Team Roles (Table 1)

Real-world implementation of these roles reduces time to action and improves outcomes.

TEAMWORK DYNAMICS IN OBSTETRIC EMERGENCIES

In obstetric emergencies like PPH, teamwork dynamics play a pivotal role. The *'zero delay' principle* is crucial, where time-sensitive decisions are taken without hierarchy-induced delays.

TABLE 1: Team members and their roles.

Team member	*Key role*
Obstetrician	Clinical lead, diagnosis and surgical intervention
Nurse	IV access, monitoring vitals, preparing medications
Anesthetist	Hemodynamic stabilization, airway management
Blood bank officer	Crossmatch and issue blood products
Support staff	Mobilize equipment, patient transfer if needed

Features of High-performance Obstetric Teams

- *Mutual trust:* Enables seamless task delegation.
- *Closed-loop communication:* Prevents miscommunication ("Oxytocin 10 IU IV given"—acknowledged by team lead).
- *Adaptive leadership:* The team leader reassesses and reprioritizes based on patient response.
- *Debriefing post-event:* Strengthens team cohesion and learning.

The use of *PPH carts, pre-labeled emergency trays,* and *PPH checklists* can dramatically reduce the time taken to initiate action, but only when the team is trained and confident in their roles.

STRUCTURED COMMUNICATION IN PPH MANAGEMENT

SBAR: A Proven Tool

The *SBAR* technique is globally recommended to facilitate concise and structured communication in emergencies:

- *S—Situation:* "This is a 26-year-old primigravida with ongoing heavy bleeding 15 minutes after delivery."
- *B—Background:* "Vaginal delivery, 39 weeks, no complications during labor."
- *A—Assessment:* "Uterus boggy, bleeding approximately 1,000 mL, BP 90/60."
- *R—Recommendation:* "Start uterotonics, prepare for possible surgical intervention."

Importance in Indian Settings

In India, where many births are conducted in resource-limited settings, the use of standardized communication tools helps avoid misinterpretations, particularly when working with staff of varying experience levels or language barriers.

Additional Communication Strategies

- Use of *PPH Emergency Codes* (e.g., Code Red)
- Laminated SBAR cards at the bedside
- Training nurses and interns in communication etiquette

LEADERSHIP AND ROLE CLARITY DURING PPH

Closed-loop Communication

Closed-loop communication involves confirming receipt and understanding of a message by repeating it back. For instance, if a team leader says, "Administer 1 gram of tranexamic acid IV now," the team member should respond, "Administering 1 gram of tranexamic acid IV now," and then confirm once it is done. This feedback loop ensures that:

- Orders are not missed or misheard.
- Tasks are tracked and completed.
- Responsibility is clear.

This method is essential during PPH, as multiple interventions occur simultaneously—fluid resuscitation, medication administration, surgical preparation, uterine massage, and blood transfusion coordination—each needing accurate execution.

SBAR Format for Communication

The SBAR (Situation, Background, Assessment, Recommendation) technique is widely advocated for structured communication in obstetric emergencies. It helps junior staff and nurses escalate concerns to senior clinicians confidently and ensures efficient information transfer.

- *Situation:* "This is a 29-year-old G2P1 who has just delivered vaginally and is bleeding profusely."
- *Background:* "She had a 3rd stage lasting over 30 minutes and was on oxytocin induction for 14 hours."
- *Assessment:* "Fundus is boggy, approximately 800 ml blood loss, no retained placenta."
- *Recommendation:* "Requesting immediate PPH protocol activation and senior obstetrician review."

SBAR reduces ambiguity and helps standardize critical communication across all levels of expertise.

Multi-disciplinary Coordination

In managing PPH, obstetricians, anesthetists, midwives, nursing staff, blood bank personnel, and sometimes interventional radiologists must synchronize their roles. Communication strategies should define:

- Primary leader of the resuscitation team.
- Defined runners for drug collection and equipment.
- Backup personnel who can take over roles when someone becomes task-saturated.

Regular verbal updates—"Blood loss is now 1300 ml, uterotonics given, preparing for surgical intervention"—allow real-time shared mental modeling among team members.

Communication Barriers

Several barriers hinder effective communication in PPH emergencies:

- Hierarchical culture where junior staff hesitate to speak up.
- Language differences or unclear accents in multicultural teams.

- Background noise in labor wards, especially during shift changes.
- Panic or cognitive overload in the face of critical maternal deterioration.

Overcoming these requires a culture of psychological safety, where all team members feel empowered to speak, alert, question, or escalate care without fear of reprisal.

Use of Communication Aids

- Whiteboards or digital displays in the delivery suite can record timelines of drug administration, estimated blood loss, and steps taken.
- Color-coded checklists and communication cards (e.g., "Blood Requested," "Balloon Tamponade Ready") help relay updates quickly and visually.
- Dedicated communication liaisons can be assigned to speak with family members, keeping them informed while avoiding distraction of clinical staff.

Communicating with Patients and Families

Even during an emergency, it is essential to:

- Reassure the patient using simple, empathetic language.
- Inform her about procedures being undertaken (e.g., "We are giving medications to help your uterus contract.")
- Keep the family updated in real-time to reduce panic.

Clear communication with patients also ensures informed consent for surgical procedures, blood transfusions, or escalation to ICU care.

Simulation Training and Drills for Team Preparedness

Simulation-based learning is a game-changer in obstetric emergencies. It allows team members to:

- Practice emergency protocols without patient risk
- Improve communication and crisis response
- Develop non-technical skills like leadership and teamwork

Types of Simulations

- *Low-fidelity drills* using mannequins for uterine massage and bimanual compression
- *High-fidelity simulations* in labor wards with real-time role play and mock scenarios
- *Unannounced drills* to test team responsiveness

Evidence

Studies show that institutions conducting *quarterly drills* have significantly *lower rates of delay in administering uterotonics* and better blood transfusion practices.

Effective Record Maintenance in PPH

Documentation in PPH is *not just for legal protection*—it is a *clinical tool* to monitor progress, communicate across shifts, and identify preventable factors.

Essential Documentation Elements

- Time of delivery and onset of bleeding
- Estimated blood loss (preferably quantified with calibrated drapes)
- Uterotonic agents used (dose/time/route)
- Vitals charted every 5–10 minutes
- Surgical interventions done
- Blood and blood product administration
- Response to treatment
- Team members involved
- Consent for procedures, especially invasive ones

Recommended Tools

- *PPH Flow Sheets* with timestamped actions
- *Checklist-based charts* for uterotonic administration
- *Color-coded records* to distinguish emergency events

Electronic health records with *real-time alerts* are being introduced in tertiary centers to facilitate better record keeping and reduce omissions.

LEGAL AND MEDICO-LEGAL IMPLICATIONS OF POOR DOCUMENTATION

Rationale for Simulation-based Training

PPH is often sudden and unpredictable, occurring in both high-risk and low-risk deliveries. While guidelines and protocols exist, the *real-world implementation* of these protocols depends heavily on the team's ability to respond under pressure. *Simulation training* helps:

- Reinforce PPH management protocols.
- Build team coordination and confidence.
- Provide a safe environment to practice rare or complex scenarios.
- Identify latent errors in the system or layout.

Just like CPR and neonatal resuscitation, obstetric emergency drills including PPH are now considered a *standard component of maternity safety programs.*

Types of Simulations

Simulations can vary depending on the resources available:

- *Low-fidelity simulations:* Using mannequins or actors to mimic blood loss, uterine atony, and team responses.

- *High-fidelity simulations:* Computerized mannequins with programmable vital signs, bleeding, and feedback systems.
- *Hybrid simulations:* Combination of virtual reality (VR) and physical components.
- *Tabletop simulations:* For administrative and interdepartmental flow testing, especially for coordination with ICU or blood bank.

Frequency and Customization of Drills

- *Monthly or quarterly drills* focusing on different PPH scenarios: uterine atony, retained placenta, surgical complications, DIC, etc.
- *Customizing scenarios* based on institutional gaps (e.g., delayed blood availability, poor communication between floors).
- Simulations should involve the *entire obstetric ecosystem*—labor room staff, anesthetists, lab technicians, porters, and blood bank staff.

Debriefing: The Core of Simulation Learning

Debriefing after simulations allows:

- Open reflection on what went right or wrong.
- Discussion of *non-technical skills* like communication, leadership, and teamwork.
- Identification of *system errors*—missing equipment, faulty suction, delay in drug availability.

The *PLUS/DELTA* method is often used: "What went well (Plus)" and "What can we change (Delta)?"

Benefits of Simulation Training

- Improves *time-to-intervention metrics* (e.g., time from diagnosis to tranexamic acid administration).
- Builds familiarity with *PPH kits, tamponade balloons,* and *massive transfusion protocols.*
- Reduces staff anxiety and improves decision-making confidence.
- Prepares junior doctors and rotating residents to act swiftly during their on-call duties.

Integration into Quality Improvement

Simulation outcomes should feed into a hospital's *clinical governance* and *audit* programs. For instance:

- If multiple drills reveal delays in accessing blood products, the hospital may redesign the transfusion protocol.
- If the team repeatedly forgets to activate the PPH emergency buzzer, this may indicate a training need or technical issue.

Simulation is not just training—it is an active *patient safety and system optimization tool.*

Challenges and Solutions

- *Time constraints:* Can be solved by integrating short "in-situ" drills during shifts.
- *Staff resistance or apathy:* Addressed through leadership endorsement and rewards.
- *Resource limitations:* Low-cost simulations using common items can still be very effective.

International Recommendations

The *World Health Organization (WHO)*, *FIGO*, and national bodies like *NHS UK* and *FOGSI* advocate for mandatory simulation training in obstetric emergencies, including PPH.

CHALLENGES IN LOW-RESOURCE SETTINGS

In rural or peripheral centers, obstacles include:
- Limited staff availability at odd hours
- Inadequate training in emergency drills
- Delayed access to blood products
- Cultural hesitation in escalating care or referring

Solutions

- *Task shifting:* Train nurses and midwives in PPH management
- *Tele-obstetrics:* Remote guidance from tertiary care
- *Portable blood loss measurement tools*
- Use of *non-pneumatic anti-shock garments (NASG)* to buy time during transfers

TECHNOLOGICAL INTERVENTIONS TO AID TEAMWORK AND DOCUMENTATION

Modern tools enhancing PPH care:
- *Mobile Apps* for PPH management algorithms (e.g., Safe Delivery App)
- *QR-coded PPH protocols* at the bedside
- *Digital dashboards* for real-time team alerts
- *Voice-to-text record maintenance* in labor rooms

Integration of *AI-enabled monitoring tools* is an emerging frontier that can support teams by flagging deviations in vitals.

RECOMMENDATIONS AND GLOBAL BEST PRACTICES

WHO Recommendations

- Establish emergency response teams in all obstetric units
- Standard operating procedures for PPH
- Drills at least every 6 months
- Document blood loss using calibrated containers, not visual estimation

FIGO and FOGSI Recommendations

- Promote early identification and bundled care
- Encourage formation of PPH audit teams
- Record keeping as a standard performance metric
- Use of uterine balloon tamponade and NASG as interim measures

ROLE OF DEBRIEFING AND AUDITS IN CONTINUOUS IMPROVEMENT

Clinical Debriefing: Learning from Experience

Clinical debriefing is a focused discussion that takes place after the management of a critical event like PPH. The goal is not to blame but to reflect, evaluate, and improve.

Key Components of a Structured Debriefing

- *What went well:* Acknowledging actions that were timely and effective boosts team morale and helps reinforce best practices.
- *What could have gone better:* Identifying missed opportunities, delays, or lapses in coordination.
- *What needs to change:* Suggestions for modifying systems, refining protocols, or improving training.
- *Who should be involved:* All members of the response team—obstetricians, anesthetists, midwives, nurses, and support staff—should be included. Multidisciplinary involvement ensures a 360-degree view of the event.

Timing

- Hot debriefs are conducted immediately after the event, often in the delivery room, while details are fresh.
- Cold debriefs are more structured and scheduled within 24–72 hours post-event. They allow emotions to settle and provide an opportunity for deeper analysis.

Benefits of Debriefing

- Enhances communication between team members.
- Reduces the risk of burnout by allowing emotional processing.

- Improves future preparedness and team coordination.
- Identifies equipment, logistic, or recordkeeping challenges.
- Promotes a culture of transparency and learning.

Simulation-based Debriefing

Increasingly, PPH simulations are integrated into maternity team training programs. These simulations are followed by debriefs where actions and decision-making processes are critically evaluated.

Simulation debriefs can help:

- *R*ehearse rare but high-risk scenarios.
- Build team reflexes and reinforce communication protocols (e.g., SBAR format).
- Identify gaps in individual knowledge and team function.

Clinical Audit: Driving Systemic Change

A clinical audit is a systematic review of care against defined criteria with the aim to improve outcomes. It is both retrospective and prospective—looking at what has occurred and what should be improved going forward.

Steps in a PPH Clinical Audit

1. Define the audit topic—e.g., time to activation of massive transfusion protocol in PPH.
2. Set criteria and standards—derived from national guidelines (e.g., WHO, FIGO, RCOG, FOGSI).
3. Collect data—from records, partographs, operation notes, transfusion slips, and team reports.
4. Compare performance with standards—identify where standards were not met.
5. Implement change—targeted training, protocol revision, or system-level upgrades.
6. Re-audit—after a defined interval to assess improvement.

Indicators often Audited in PPH Cases

- Time to diagnosis and response initiation.
- Volume of blood lost vs estimated.
- Time to involvement of senior staff.
- Blood product usage and appropriateness.
- Compliance with WHO PPH care bundle.
- Documentation quality and completeness.

Root Cause Analysis (RCA) in Adverse Outcomes

In severe cases with maternal near-miss or mortality, Root Cause Analysis (RCA) is mandated in many tertiary institutions and teaching hospitals. RCA involves a thorough investigation into underlying causes—not just clinical but organizational, human factors, and systemic issues.

Example of RCA findings in PPH:

- Lack of availability of uterotonic drugs.
- Failure to escalate care due to hierarchical communication barriers.
- Delay in shifting patient to operation theater.
- Miscommunication between blood bank and labor ward.
- Incomplete documentation leading to medicolegal vulnerability.

RCA often recommends structured changes such as:

- Re-training staff on emergency response.
- Updating the PPH kit and ensuring accessibility.
- Redesigning the handover sheet to include bleeding risk.

Learning Health System (LHS) Model

In high-performing maternity units, audits and debriefings contribute to a Learning Health System—one that continuously collects data, analyzes it, learns from it, and integrates improvements into everyday clinical care.

Features of an LHS Model Applied to PPH

- *D*igital dashboards tracking PPH events.
- Monthly morbidity and mortality (M&M) meetings.
- Quarterly reviews of blood loss patterns and transfusion rates.
- Staff newsletters highlighting lessons from recent events.

Role of Leadership in Institutionalizing Feedback

Leadership plays a key role in ensuring debriefing and audit mechanisms are:

- Non-punitive
- Consistent
- Well-documented
- Result-oriented

Department heads must:

- Encourage open conversations.
- Allocate time and space for debriefings.
- Empower staff to speak up during audits.
- Protect team members from blame while ensuring accountability.

Challenges in Implementation

Despite the proven value of debriefing and audit, several barriers exist:

- Time constraints in busy labor wards.
- Lack of documentation or inadequate recordkeeping hampers accurate review.
- Fear of legal consequences inhibits open discussion.
- Hierarchical systems discourage junior staff from offering input.

To overcome these, institutional support, protected time, confidentiality, and anonymized data reviews are critical.

Linking Audit to Policy Change

A single PPH case may reveal the need for broader institutional or regional changes:

- Creation of regional blood bank networking.
- Introduction of visual aids for early estimation of blood loss.
- Mandating antenatal risk assessment documentation.
- Updating pre-filled PPH management checklists.

Clinical audit findings should not stay within the team but be escalated to hospital administration and health authorities when necessary.

Global and National Examples

- *UK NHS:* The MBRRACE-UK Confidential Enquiries publish annual reports that rely heavily on audits and debriefs from individual maternal deaths.
- *India (FOGSI):* Encourages confidential enquiry forms post-maternal mortality for learning and audit, especially for preventable causes like PPH.
- *WHO Recommendations:* Promote maternal death surveillance and response (MDSR) systems as standard practice in all countries.

Digital Tools Supporting Debrief and Audit

Emerging digital tools now support real-time feedback and debriefing:

- Mobile-based audit apps allowing instant upload of findings.
- AI-driven dashboards analyzing PPH incidence and response times.
- Electronic PPH checklists capturing timestamps for key interventions.

Digital integration ensures timely feedback, larger data pooling, and evidence-based improvements on a broader scale.

CONCLUSION

Managing PPH effectively is not the burden of a single doctor or nurse—it is a *team-driven, communication-reliant,* and *documentation-dependent* process.

Every second matters, and every action needs to be recorded, communicated, and coordinated.

The convergence of *clinical readiness, non-technical skills*, and *robust record systems* is what ultimately saves lives. As India marches toward improving maternal health outcomes under *LaQshya* and *Surakshit Matritva Abhiyan*, embedding these principles is essential.

SUGGESTED READING

1. FIGO Safe Motherhood and Newborn Health Committee. Management of postpartum hemorrhage. Int J Gynaecol Obstet. 2022;157(2):198-206.
2. Knight M, Bunch K, Tuffnell D, Patel R, Shakespeare J, Kotnis R, et al. Saving Lives, Improving Mothers' Care—Lessons learned to inform maternity care from the UK and Ireland Confidential Enquiries into Maternal Deaths and Morbidity 2019-21. Oxford: National Perinatal Epidemiology Unit, University of Oxford; 2023.
3. Main EK, Cape V, Abreo A, Vasher J, Woods A, Carpenter A, et al. Reduction of severe maternal morbidity from hemorrhage using a state perinatal quality collaborative. Am J Obstet Gynecol. 2021;224(3):278.e1-278.e11.
4. Mhyre JM, D'Oria R, Hameed AB, Lappen JR, Holley SL, Hunter SK, et al. The maternal early warning criteria: a proposal from the National Partnership for Maternal Safety. Obstet Gynecol. 2020;133(5):843-52.
5. Pandey A, Shrestha N, Acharya N, Adhikari S. Documentation and outcomes in postpartum hemorrhage: a retrospective study in a tertiary hospital. Int J Gynaecol Obstet. 2023;160(1):86-92.
6. Say L, Chou D, Gemmill A, Tunçalp Ö, Moller AB, Daniels JD, et al. Global causes of maternal death: a WHO systematic analysis. Lancet Glob Health. 2022;10(3):e388-e395.
7. Sheikh S, Qureshi RN, Khowaja AR, Hoodbhoy Z, Zaidi S, Sawchuck D, et al. Teamwork and communication in PPH management: a qualitative analysis from a simulation-based study in Pakistan. BMJ Open. 2021;11(4):e043974.
8. World Health Organization. WHO recommendations: Uterotonics for the prevention of postpartum haemorrhage. Geneva: WHO; 2020.